Chronic Fatigue Syndrome and Fibromyalgia

From F.I.N.E.

(Frustrated, Irritated, Nauseated, Exhausted)

to

Feeling Better

**Nancy Fowler
Lisa Ball**

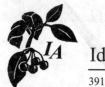

Idyll Arbor, Inc.

39129 264th Ave SE, Enumclaw, WA 98022 (360) 825-7797

ISBN: 9781882883684

Printed in the United States of America

Library of Congress Cataloging-in-Publication Data

Fowler, Nancy, 1942-
  Chronic fatigue syndrome and fibromyalgia : from F.I.N.E. (frustrated, irritated, nauseated, exhausted) to feeling better / Nancy Fowler, Lisa Ball.
       p. cm.
  Includes bibliographical references and index.
  ISBN 978-1-882883-68-4 (alk. paper)
  1. Chronic fatigue syndrome--Popular works. 2. Fibromyalgia--Popular works. I. Ball, Lisa, 1960- II. Title.
  RB150.F37F677 2010
  616'.0478--dc22

                                                              2009038620

This book is respectfully dedicated to all who suffer from this illness and to one who no longer does.

In Loving Memory
Dyanne Comeau, August 16, 2001

The heart that cares remembers
With the passing of the years,
The memories created
By our laughter, by our tears.
The heart that cares remembers
The secrets that we shared,
The dreams we had, the trust we earned,
The friends who showed they cared.
The heart that cares remembers
Because often we lose touch
With those whose lives once touched ours,
They still mean so very much.
The heart that cares remembers
When two strangers became two friends,
They forged a bond that will endure
On that you can depend.
The heart that cares remembers
And misses what used to be,
It mourns that loss, but this I know:
We'll always be friends…you and me.

There are no such things as incurables;
there are only things for which man has not found a cure.
— Bernard M. Baruch

CONTENTS

FOREWORD

The conditions discussed in this book are mystifying, exasperating, often debilitating, misunderstood, misdiagnosed, scary, confusing, expensive, anything-but-routine, and *real*. Our hope is to provide you with common sense solutions and answers to questions in everyday language that is easy to understand.

It should be noted that many people believe that fibromyalgia and chronic fatigue syndrome are two different illnesses. It may be possible to have fibromyalgia and not have CFS. Or to have CFS without having fibromyalgia. Or to have *both* fibromyalgia and CFS. Even worse there is another name that many people use to describe the condition, chronic fatigue and immune dysfunction syndrome (CFIDS). The immune deficiency part is in there somewhere, too. See how confusing it can be?

As you can imagine, the confusion may (understandably) lead to a missed diagnosis. We feel that by referring to the two different but remarkably similar illnesses as one we are reducing any confusion encountered without causing harm.

What we hope to instill in the reader is this: if a person says they are sick or in pain *believe* them! They know how they feel. And if you have this illness, NEVER DOUBT YOURSELF. What you are feeling is real and not in your imagination. Pay attention to your body, and *do not* be tempted to attribute all of your health problems to this illness. Having CFS or fibromyalgia doesn't mean you can't get another illness such as cancer, heart disease, or diabetes.

Throughout this book you will encounter these abbreviations that you may be unfamiliar with:

FM — Fibromyalgia

CFS — Chronic Fatigue Syndrome

CFIDS — Chronic Fatigue and Immune Dysfunction Syndrome

PWF/C — Person with Fibromyalgia/CFS

PWTT — Person with "The Thief" in their life (The Thief is how we refer to our illness.)

DISCLAIMER:

Please understand that we DO NOT ENDORSE any particular treatment, medication, or practitioner, and we strongly urge you to consult your doctor before starting any treatment regimen.

We also want you to know that we care about you, and we know and understand all that you are enduring. Please be assured — you can survive and *live* with this illness. Don't let yourself become a victim to it.

Thank you.

Nancy Fowler
Lisa Ball

ACKNOWLEDGEMENTS

We wish to thank and acknowledge the following people and institutions for their invaluable and ongoing assistance in our quest to promote awareness and provide information about this devastating illness. Without their help and support this book would not be possible.

Thank you to: The Seacoast Chapter Support Group of the National CFIDS Foundation. We have learned something from each and every one of you, and you are all very special to us. Very special thanks to Beverly, Shirley, Rebecca, Carol, and of course, John. You are, without a doubt, the ABSOLUTE GREATEST!

From Lisa: To my husband, Greg and my daughter, Cassie: Thank you for giving me the love and strength I need to carry on each and every day. I thank you for your never-ending faith in me, your patience, and for providing me with much of my material. I love you both dearly. Mostly I want to thank you, Lord, for giving me a serving heart so I can listen, encourage, and help those in need who are suffering from this debilitating illness.

Last, but not least, thank you to Nancy who is my rock, my strength, and my dearest friend. Without her love, support, and organizational skills this book would not have become a reality.

From Nancy: To my husband, Rick, my son Fred, my B.F.F., Shirley Paine, and most of all to my "Sunshine," my grand-daughter,

Rachel, who brought the sun back into my life. I love and cherish you all. Lastly, thank you most of all to Lisa. This book was her idea, and without her encouragement, suggestions, and superb editorial skills this book would not have made it past the "we should write a book" stage. I couldn't ask for a better friend or cheerleader. Love ya, Lisa!

We could not possibly forget the ongoing support and help of Frisbie Memorial Hospital in Rochester, NH; Wentworth Douglass Hospital in Dover, NH; the Rochester Elks Lodge; Gail Kansky, president of the National CFIDS Foundation; and last but not least, THANK YOU to Tom Blaschko, Mary Kieffer, Sand Swenby, MD, at Idyll Arbor for having faith in us. We truly appreciate all you have done for us.

P.S. There are undoubtedly others who deserve our thanks, but unfortunately, "fibro-fog" has struck again. It's not that we aren't grateful for your help — we are, and we love you. We just forgot (temporarily) who you are and what you did to help us. Please forgive us and accept our most heartfelt apologies. As you know, it REALLY isn't our fault!

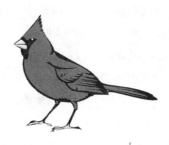

INTRODUCTION

A strong, positive mental attitude will create more
miracles than any wonder drug.
— Patricia Neal, American actress

Her mother and father were once very much in love, but over time their feelings changed. Mother was the strong one. Her goal in life was to make her husband a "success." Daddy tried, but failed to meet Mother's expectations.

He was the proud father of two girls, and Daddy believed, much to Mother's consternation, that girls should have a proper education. The elder daughter rebelled and refused, whining and complaining at the prospect. The younger daughter was prettier, smarter, more charming, and the apple of her daddy's eye. She yearned for knowledge, reveling in the learning experience, and Daddy was only too happy to oblige his little girl.

As a child, though, she always felt she was different. She felt like a monster. She refused to dine with the rest of the family because she was afraid that she would not use the knife and fork as other people did. She lived in fear of meeting children because she was afraid of not pleasing them, and so retreated into her very own "dream world" where she was

1

always the heroine. This was her way of escaping from a world in which she felt uncomfortable.

As she grew up she became more beautiful. Tall and willowy, she had a beautiful figure, silky, wavy, chestnut brown hair, and gray eyes. She attracted the attention of many young men and she would receive several proposals of marriage, all of which she would refuse.

She became a woman of strong passions, was rarely given to praise, and didn't know the meaning of forgive and forget, for that was not part of her being. She had little tolerance for opinions other than her own. She was censorious and had an enormous ego. Everyone had to meet her expectations.

When striving to make a decision she would seek out competent advice, garner all the facts, and upon reaching a conclusion, she would not change her mind or stray from the course she had set.

She did not tolerate delays, nor would she tolerate any opposition to her decisions. She had no patience for those who acted without knowing the whys and wherefores of their actions. She had no use for anyone who had knowledge for the sake of knowledge or knowledge that led to no useful action. In her mind, the greatest sins were for a woman to be "only enthusiastic" (all words and no action) and for a man to be "unbusiness-like."

Yet, she possessed infinite compassion and a true, honest love for the unfortunate, the sick, the injured, and the displaced. Her unceasing goal was to love and serve those people. She was extremely modest and shied away from the praise and honors that came her way. She constantly strived for perfection, which she felt she never attained, and was capable of deep self-pity and feelings of martyrdom.

She inspired great loyalty and devotion, but was also manipulative, and keenly aware of her power and influence. She actually worked a close friend to death and then castigated him without mercy as he lie dying; yet the man's last words were an apology to her because he felt he had failed her.

She admitted to hearing voices four times in her life. Each incident occurred after a period of extreme emotional and psychological stress that was marked by personal disappointment, extreme self-doubt, and deep depression. After hearing the voices, she felt a strong desire to accomplish something important, which lead to her devotion to her work and the sense of fulfillment it brought.

She was asked to go to war and she did. She brought order where there was chaos, and hope where there was none. She elicited such feelings of love and devotion that one soldier said that he was "struck with the desire to just kiss her shadow as she passed." So competent and effective was she that the death rate was drastically reduced in her first few weeks of service. Over the next year the mortality rate dropped even further. In effect, it was she who won the war — not the Allies.

But the war took a huge toll on her and she returned from the killing fields a very ill woman. She suffered from extreme fatigue, palpitations, hair loss, difficulty breathing, fainting spells, rheumatism, irritable bowel, nausea, depression, and many other troubling symptoms. The illness lasted the rest of her life.

Today they might call her illness Gulf War Syndrome. They might call it fibromyalgia or CFS. Back then they called it Crimean Fever.

"She" was Florence Nightingale. And if anybody understood *pain*, it was Florence, because she experienced pain, either physical or psychological, for most of her life. Florence Nightingale's birthday is May 12, and that is why that date was chosen as Fibromyalgia Awareness Day.

The purpose behind any day of awareness is to educate and inform. We want to educate you about chronic pain. We want to help you understand it and to help you win your battle against pain. We want to help you and your loved ones to cope with and thereby defeat it. We may not be able to provide all the answers or solutions, but we are sure going to try. We are, or have at some time, been in your shoes. We know, we understand, and we care.

Pain is subjective. The only person who knows the pain is the person who owns it — the person experiencing it. A description of pain could be "whatever the person experiencing it says it is. It is as mild or severe, lasts as briefly or long, and is relieved or not relieved by whatever the person experiencing it says."

But it is *not* just the person experiencing pain who is affected. Those who love and care for that person are also affected. They want to help but don't know how. They fear touching, they fear holding, they fear loving, because those actions may cause more pain. Sometimes loving caregivers begin to distance themselves emotionally because they're afraid that they, too, will eventually be hurt.

A cold, vicious circle of pain begins to develop and all parties begin to hurt. Being a circle, it can't be determined where the pain began, nor when — or if — it will ever end. We want to try to break that circle.

Everyone *needs* to love and be loved, and everyone *needs* loving touch. Open, honest communication is needed in order to replace that vicious circle of pain with another circle, one of love and compassion. Only then will that once cold, vicious circle begin to feel safe and comforting, like another circle — one that is known as a hug. A gentle hug.

In case you're feeling that you're alone in this battle, or that only ordinary people like yourself get this illness, here's a list of people you may have heard of that know and understand what you are experiencing, because they also have this illness.

Michelle Akers — member of the United States Women's National Soccer Team, Olympic gold medalist, and member of the National Soccer Hall of Fame

Charles Darwin — English naturalist who developed the theory of evolution by natural selection

Amy Peterson — Olympic speed skater

Keith Jarrett — Jazz musician

Blake Edwards — American film director, screenwriter, and producer

James Garner — Actor

Morgan Fairchild — Actress

Alana Stuart — Actress, former model, and ex-wife of George Hamilton and Rod Stewart

Kim Gallagher — Two-time Olympic medalist in track and field

Laura Hillenbrand — Author of best-selling book, *Seabiscuit: An American Legend*

Susan Harris Witt — TV comedy writer and producer (Soap, Benson, The Golden Girls, Empty Nest)

Devin Starlanyl, MD — Author of best-selling book, *Fibromyalgia and Chronic Myofascial Pain — a Survivor's Manual*

Alfred Nobel — Inventor of dynamite; originated the Nobel Prize

Grahame Cheney — Australian light welterweight boxer and 1988 Olympic silver medalist

Gilda Radner — Emmy Award winning actress and comedienne

Andrés Segovia — Spanish classical guitarist

It kind of gives you hope and inspiration, doesn't it?

We've also included a number of stories throughout the book about everyday people who are dealing with this illness. You may recognize yourself in some of their stories. The names have been changed and we've taken some poetic license to protect privacy, but the basic truths have been left untouched.

1
NAME THAT PAIN

It is possible that I am more seriously ill than my
doctors think. The pain will not go away.
— Alfred Nobel

"What's in a name?" "A name has many faces." Many names have been given to our pain over the years. Some may have come from a medical professional or perhaps from your grandmother. Let's see how many names have been bestowed upon this *one* illness:

Fibromyalgia

Chronic Fatigue Syndrome (CFS)

Chronic Fatigue and Immune Dysfunction Syndrome (CFIDS)

Chronic Immune Activation Syndrome (CIAS)

Fibrositis

Fibromyositis

Myalgic Encephalomyelitis

Post Viral Fatigue Syndrome

Myofascial Pain Syndrome

Galloping Rheumatism

Rheumatism

Tension Myalgia

Muscular Rheumatism

Myalgia

Chronic Rheumatism

Pressure Point Syndrome

Muscle Hardening

Psychogenic Rheumatism

Soft Tissue Rheumatism

Occupational Myalgia

Trigger Point Syndrome

Myofascial Pain Dysfunction

Growing Pains

Cumulative Trauma Disorder

Occupational Overuse Strain

Gulf War Syndrome

Nightingale Syndrome

Chronic Pain Syndrome

Multiple Chemical Sensitivities (MCS)

Cytomegalovirus (CMV)

Chronic Epstein-Barr Virus (CEBV)

Yuppie Flu

Crimean Fever

Chronic Mononucleosis

These names all refer to the *same* illness, one that many people DO NOT BELIEVE EXISTS and over which confusion and debate continue to rage. The most important and unfortunate part of all this confusion is that the patient can become lost and almost secondary to the debate.

Throughout this book we occasionally refer to fibromyalgia/CFS as "The Thief." After much thought, we settled on this euphemism as the least offensive and most descriptive term for a most offensive and profane illness. The Thief is an appropriate designation because it does, indeed, steal from you and your loved ones.

Think of your body and brain as a large, intricate, and well-guarded bank safe. Now think of your illness as a master thief, one who has somehow snuck past the guards, defeated your security system, cracked the safe, and now controls every aspect of your life. *EVERY ASPECT.* The Thief now controls you financially, physically, emotionally, socially, and sexually, and life as you knew it will never be the same. One day this fact will hit you. On the day it hit me, I made a conscious decision to fight my illness by accepting it and not denying what was happening to my body, my brain, and my life.

The patient doesn't care *what* it's called. We only know we're in pain: confused, feeling frightened and alone, mistrusting everyone — family, friends, medical personnel, and, most of all, ourselves.

Because of these feelings of helplessness and hopelessness, and the perception that no one cares, believes, or understands what we are going through, many patients experience a secondary depression. Many consider suicide. Some even attempt it — and worse, some succeed.

PATTI

Patti is well loved, energetic, gracious, and generous to a fault. If you needed help you could go to Patti. If she wasn't able to help you, she knew who could. Soft spoken and determined, she wouldn't stop until she got you the help you needed. No one was ever turned away.

But Patti had a well-guarded secret — she was in pain. No one ever knew that *she* needed help. Something inside of her would not let her seek help for herself, yet help was what she desperately needed.

People would tell her how beautiful she was, how great she looked. "What's your secret for staying so young?" they would ask. Patti just smiled and thanked them for the compliment. No one ever guessed how much pain she was in. No one could know how much pain those well-meant compliments caused. Yeah, she looked good — very good. She didn't *look* sick. None of the doctors she had been to could find anything wrong with her. So she thought, "Maybe I'm imagining all this pain. Maybe it's all in my head. Maybe I'm crazy."

This went on for days, weeks, months — years passed until finally Patti decided she'd had enough. She couldn't bear the pain any longer. Soon it would be over. No more pain. No more secrets.

Soon it would be over...so soon. Patti closed her eyes. Sleep was near, and she began to feel at peace. Soon the pain would be gone. What a pleasant thought...sleep...m-m-m-m-m, ah-h-h-h-...sleep...so nice...so...but, WAIT!

What is all that noise? And those bright lights hurt her eyes. She heard people yelling — why were they yelling at her? Why were they making all that horrid noise? She wanted to go to sleep — to the place where she felt no pain. But they wouldn't let her! DAMN THEM! DAMN, DAMN, DAMN!

Then, the realization of what was happening dawned on her. Patti began to shake violently, uncontrollably. Tears began to flow and wouldn't stop. "Oh, my God! My God, my God! *What* have I *done*? Oh my God! Oh, no-o-o-o-o!" Her voice rose to a keening wail.

Suddenly, Patti was grateful. Grateful for the pain — grateful she could feel anything at all. *Grateful to be alive.* She understood the everlasting pain her death would have caused to those she loved and who loved her — her husband, her children, her family, and friends. She vowed she would make it up to them, to herself, and to God, for she had almost succeeded in throwing her life away.

It was a long, difficult, and sometimes humiliating journey back for Patti. But she made it. She is now a much stronger woman and a source of inspiration and admiration for all who know her. Yes, she still has pain, but now she knows her pain is real and can be controlled.

People still come to Patti for help with their problems and she gives it gladly and with love. She no longer doubts herself. She is a self-assured, confident woman, capable of giving and receiving love and understanding, and the ability to instill these traits in those who seek her help. She can spot the signs of someone in trouble (as she was) and she will quietly and unobtrusively take that person under her wing. She is a valuable asset to our support group.

2
MEET "THE THIEF"

*...it's stupid to call it Chronic Fatigue Syndrome. It
should be called the forever dead syndrome.*
— Keith Jarrett, jazz musician

Am I crazy?
Am I imagining things?
Is what I'm feeling real?

◊ ◊ ◊

Then your doctor makes the diagnosis and your mind is in a whirl.
You have a million more questions.

Are you sure?
Why me?
Who gets it?
How did I get it?
How long will I have it?
Will I become disabled?

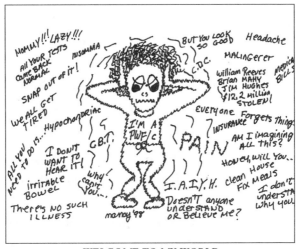

WELCOME TO MY WORLD
(A look at life through the eyes of a PWF/C)

Can I still work?

Should I still work?

Will I need to go to the hospital?

Will I need to go to a nursing home?

Is it fatal?

Is it contagious?

Can it be cured?

How is it treated?

What tests are done?

How can the doctor tell I have it?

What are the symptoms?

You are afraid of the possible answers. You don't know where to start, yet, strangely, you also feel happy and relieved. A name has finally been put to your miseries. Your symptoms are *real*, not a figment of your imagination. You're *not* a lazy hypochondriac with the beginning signs of Alzheimer's. *YOU ARE NOT GOING CRAZY.* What a relief!

And now you want to know:

What can I do to help myself?

WHAT'S NEXT?

We will attempt to answer your questions and to describe this confusing illness. The answers will be full of "definite ifs and maybes." This illness leaves you a changed person. It comes and goes — OR — maybe it will be constant. You may be mildly affected — OR — you may be severely affected. And there is no way to predict just *how* you will be affected.

Some people claim to have been cured of CFS. Oh, that would be so nice. *IF* it were true! It's our opinion that those people are most likely in a remission — a nice, long remission.

In 2006, we cheered when the National CFIDS Foundation of Needham, Massachusetts, an excellent source for information about CFS and related diseases, announced that a cause of CFS may be a zoonotic virus called Parainfluenza Virus-5, also known as Simian Virus-5. This long-awaited news was announced in their quarterly magazine, *The Forum* and though it answered a lot of questions, it raised many as well. It proved that CFS and fibromyalgia are *not* the same illness, even though the symptoms are frighteningly and strikingly similar. And while there was no mention of a virus being the cause of fibromyalgia or other related diseases, it may turn out that these CFS-like illnesses have the same or very similar cause.

The reason the news was met with such excitement is because before you can find a cure for a disease, you must first find the cause. If the disease is caused by a virus, the illness is probably contagious. The very nature of a virus allows it to enter the body and lie dormant for years until it is "awakened" and starts to spread throughout the body, wreaking havoc with your health. The illness itself is not fatal. However, secondary effects such as reactions to medications, your body's reactions to stress, society's reaction to your illness, how you view your illness and life, and of course, the mindless, bureaucratic machinations of the American health care system and your HMO can be harmful, maybe even fatal, as we will show you later.

Diagnosis is often made with great difficulty, and depends on which medical specialist you choose to consult.

If you see a rheumatologist, the diagnosis will likely be fibromyalgia. When your rheumatologist reaches a diagnosis it is because:

- Other illnesses have been ruled out by doing a complete, comprehensive medical history and conducting appropriate medical testing.
- Pain was felt in at least 11 of 18 specific points when the experienced practitioner palpated those areas.
- Pain has been present at least three months in all four quadrants of the body.
- Blood test results are within normal limits (WNL).

If you see an allergist or immunologist, the diagnosis will be multiple chemical sensitivities (MCS). When a diagnosis of MCS has been reached it is because:

- Other illnesses have been ruled out by doing a complete, comprehensive medical history and conducting appropriate medical testing.
- Appropriate bloods tests have been performed, such as a complete blood count (CBC) with differential, sedimentation rate, and tests for Lyme disease, thyroid function, Epstein-Barr virus, AIDS, mononucleosis, HHV-6, arthritis profile, and cytomegalovirus.

- Possible allergies or sensitivities to foods, environmental allergens, and medications have been assessed.
- Pain and fatigue have been present for at least three months.

If you go to an infectious disease specialist, the diagnosis will be chronic fatigue syndrome (CFS). This diagnosis is reached in much the same manner as the other specialties, with fatigue being the primary, presenting complaint.

While no specific test confirms the diagnosis, tests should be done nevertheless. It is our firm belief, however, that any testing performed should be absolutely *necessary* and *pertinent*. Unnecessary tests or those with borderline relevancy tend to be expensive, painful, and worrisome to the patient. A whole list of "what ifs" begin to build in the patient's mind. Worry leads to stress and stress can lead to an exacerbation or "flare" of symptoms. Basically, at this stage, tests are done to rule out other illnesses such as:

multiple sclerosis (MS)
mononucleosis (Mono)
parasitic infections
rheumatoid arthritis
systemic lupus erythematosus (Lupus)
cytomegalovirus (CMV)
toxoplasmosis
Lyme disease
acquired immune deficiency syndrome (AIDS)
coxsackievirus
chronic hepatitis (hepatitis B; hepatitis C)
human herpes virus 6 (HHV-6)
Epstein-Barr virus (EBV)
lymphoma

thyroid disease

diabetes

major primary depression

Raynaud's phenomena

cancer

To be fair, the number and variety of symptoms experienced by victims of chronic fatigue syndrome and fibromyalgia overlap many other diseases. Multiple sclerosis and carpal tunnel syndrome both produce numbness and tingling sensations. So does The Thief in some people.

So it's no wonder that some medical professionals doubt the existence of CFS and fibromyalgia, especially when you add the fact that neither illness has a definitive diagnostic test or treatment. To further confuse and complicate matters, each patient has differing symptoms and responses to treatments.

If a disease or condition presents in the same way, affects each patient in the same manner, and responds the same to the same treatment, well then, life is a little easier. But with these illnesses, all bets are off.

Many victims of The Thief blame every health problem they have on it. This is a *huge* mistake, one that can be very dangerous. Every victim of chronic fatigue syndrome or fibromyalgia would do well to remember that just because they have this type of chronic disease does not mean that they can't get cancer, heart disease, diabetes, or other serious illness. *All of us* must be keenly aware of our body and its normal functioning so that, when something abnormal occurs, the event can be examined and treated further if necessary.

DYANNE

Lisa's cousin, Dyanne, was the classic Type-A personality for all of her 47 years. She loved life and people, worked hard, played hard, and demanded a lot from life. She was a go-getter. She was successful professionally, starting her own business as a computer consultant for accounting software. About the only thing she failed at was finding someone to share her life with, someone who deserved her and would appreciate her. Just when she would begin to feel, "Ah, this is THE ONE!" something would happen and the relationship would end, her hopes of starting a family dashed once again.

Dyanne suffered from "growing pains" as a child, and these pains continued to be a problem throughout her life. Living in New England, with its ever-changing weather became very difficult for her. Because of this, Dyanne decided to take a trip out west to Phoenix to see what life had to offer there. Once more, she fell in love. This time it was with Arizona's landscape and weather. It didn't take long for her to establish herself and feel like a native.

Dyanne began work on an accounting program for the Air Force and was soon also working with cadets in the ROTC program. She loved it — and they loved her. She won their love and respect easily, and in many ways the young cadets became the children she never had. She talked about them often, and, when she did, her eyes would light up and her face would glow. They almost made her forget her pain. They *did* make it bearable. And she in turn made life for "her" cadets a little better.

Dyanne was good at many things, but at one thing in particular — she was especially good at denying her pain and ignoring warning signs. She knew better, but she always felt she had a good excuse.

Dyanne had been battling a painful, localized skin infection that became progressively worse over nearly a week's time. She was running a fever, had the chills, and was suffering intense pain. The infection was becoming systemic.

Yet, once again, she put her needs on hold. Her cadets were holding a banquet that night and she felt she must attend. During the banquet, Dyanne's condition worsened, despite the medications and ice packs she used to try to alleviate the pain.

She called her HMO and described her symptoms, asking for permission to go to the emergency room. Her HMO refused her request and advised her to see her primary physician on Monday. Dyanne was upset and begged for permission to go to the ER that night, but again, her request was denied.

Although she felt lousy, Dyanne felt she had no choice other than to wait. But by now the infection was spreading throughout her body and because of CFS, her immune system was too weak to fight it.

On Monday, when Dyanne didn't answer her phone, a friend came by to check on her. Dyanne was found comatose, her color gray and her vital signs diminishing. She was rushed to the hospital where she died three days later.

The infection won. The loss of Dyanne was deeply felt, both by the family she was born into and the one she cared for and nurtured — her cadets.

Dyanne's story offers many important points that we want you to remember:

1. Pay attention to your body; it gives you clues when something is wrong. It's up to you to listen and do something about it. Your body is constantly at work trying to keep itself well.

2. Don't ignore warning signs. With this illness the immune system becomes compromised and infections can develop and take over much faster than in someone with a healthy immune system.

3. Get advice from emergency room personnel before talking to your HMO.

4. Make sure someone knows you're ill so that somebody can check up on you, especially if you live alone.

5. Sometimes one or two days can make a difference.

6. You WILL be missed when you are gone.

While Dyanne was too late in seeking help for her condition, in other cases patients may seek help in the emergency room but, because symptoms can be vague and after running tests doctors can find no specific diagnosis, they are sometimes reassured and sent home.

A female member of our support group made several trips to the ER over a period of time with painful and frightening chest pain. Each time, she was sent home with a diagnosis of anxiety attack. She began to doubt herself, and the next time she had chest pain she ignored it.

It was only when the pain became unbearable, when she was (almost) sure that she was not experiencing another "anxiety attack" that she again made the familiar trek to the emergency room where she was swiftly admitted to the coronary care unit with a diagnosis of myocardial infarction (heart attack).

One can only wonder if this had happened to a man whether he would have received the same dismissive treatment initially. While a man experiencing chest pains is usually taken seriously and treated aggressively, a woman experiencing the same type of pain is sometimes dismissed with a pat on the head and a diagnosis of "anxiety." Part of this difference came from the belief that women don't have heart attacks. That belief has changed during the past 10 years and women are now taken more seriously when they have heart attack symptoms. After all women are usually more in tune with their bodies and are more likely to seek help when they feel something is wrong.

We urge *everyone* to listen to your body and forget the behavior of others. Ignoring your body's warning signals can prove to be fatal, especially for people with a compromised immune system due to CFS, AIDS, or other conditions. In these people, an infection can spread unchecked throughout the body in no time at all. And there is no cure for death. Dead is dead.

If you have the "flu" or you have overworked your muscles, you will feel achy and have pain. The Thief can make you feel the same way.

Those headaches may be due to hormonal changes; or maybe you need eyeglasses or an eyeglass prescription change. Then again, maybe it's The Thief. Get to your doctor or optometrist and check it out.

If you take certain medications or have poor dietary habits you may experience Irritable Bowel Syndrome (IBS). Then again, maybe it's The Thief.

Maybe your premenstrual syndrome and painful periods are caused by The Thief. Or maybe you have a serious OB/GYN problem.

You get the idea. If you get nothing else from this book, please get this: PAY ATTENTION TO YOUR BODY AND ITS WARNING SIGNALS!

Many of us with CFS have learned to keep a health journal. The information you record in your journal will undoubtedly become valuable to you at some point. It can be used as a point of reference or comparison when health problems arise. It will help you to become more in tune with your body's normal function so you will be alerted to potentially dangerous changes.

With the often-complex symptoms, treatments, poor memory, and impaired cognitive abilities that accompany our illness, we *cannot* rely on our recollections where our health is concerned. Your journal will prove more reliable than your memory.

When recording your symptoms, do not discount such variables as weather conditions, any stressors in your life, your day-to-day activity level, the food you eat, and any medications you take. All are very important parts of the whole picture.

Your doctor will appreciate your taking an active interest and will certainly find the information you record helpful in planning your care. In addition to your journal, you may find it helpful to use a "body map" to help you accurately record exactly where you are feeling pain. You'll find a body map just like the one your doctor uses and a sample daily diary page in the Appendix. We urge you to make as many copies as you need.

3
THE SYMPTOMS

Every patient carries her or his own doctor inside.
— Albert Schweitzer

When preparing to deal with the symptoms that you may be experiencing, our advice is simple and direct: the best defense is a better offense.

Treat the worst or most troublesome symptoms first and treat them as they occur. I adhere to the KISS philosophy, or Keep It Simple, Stupid. Please don't misunderstand. I'm not calling *you* stupid. I'm simply urging you to keep things simple and uncomplicated.

You may have heard of Elizabeth Kenny, also known as Sister Kenny. Ms. Kenny was a truly amazing woman who lived in the Australian outback at the time of a rather large outbreak of infantile paralysis (polio) in the early 1900s. She had no formal medical training as a nurse but found herself in the position of being the only help available to minister to the health care needs of those stricken with that crippling virus.

Sister Kenny begged medical professionals in the urban areas for help but the doctors were fighting the same battle and had no one to spare. They promised to come to her aid as soon as possible. Dismayed and discouraged, she asked what she could do to help her patients. She was told, "Treat the symptoms as best as you can."

Sister Kenny became a good nurse, relying on her abundance of good sense. She stuck to the basics like warm, moist compresses for muscle pain and exercising the limbs to prevent atrophy. Her success rate was remarkable, and her dedication and common sense saved many from polio's crippling effects. When medical professionals finally arrived to help, they were astounded by her achievements. When asked how she managed to achieve such amazing results, Sister Kenny seemed baffled by the question and merely answered, "I treated the symptoms." Seems like Sister Kenny observed the KISS philosophy also.

The broad range of symptoms associated with chronic fatigue syndrome or fibromyalgia serve to confound and confuse anyone who makes an honest effort to understand them. These symptoms may come and go (wax and wane) or they may be constant. Treatment is usually aimed at relief of the symptoms.

When you experience an exacerbation, or "flare" of your symptoms, you *must* gain control over those symptoms. Treat your worst symptoms first, or you risk a domino effect. By controlling your most troubling, fire-of-the-moment symptoms, you will be more likely to keep control of your lesser symptoms. Being unable to control your symptoms leads to stress, and stress is something you must avoid whenever possible. In nursing, this is what is known as a "Care Plan." Your Care Plan is a plan of action you need to take to alleviate your problem symptoms.

In order to gain or regain control over your pain you must realize that it's *your* pain. You own it. Only you know what works and what doesn't

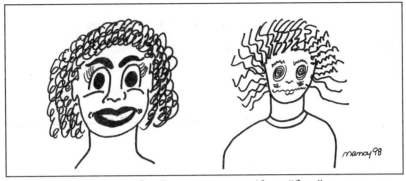

Before a "flare"   *After a "flare"*

work for you. You are the expert, so take charge of your life! Others can help you, but only you can tell them how.

Before we go much further, I want to say a few things about pain. Pain serves a very useful purpose. Pain tells us when something's wrong with our body. Pain tells us to slow down and take care of ourselves before it is too late. For example, if we didn't experience the pain of a broken foot, we would proceed in our activities not knowing anything was wrong, causing further injury and eventual incapacitation. When you burn yourself, the pain tells you to remove yourself from the heat source before you are incinerated. Pain is not considered to be an expected or usual state.

The pain inflicted by The Thief is usually described as hot and burning or as painful knots in the muscles. To further describe what chronic fatigue syndrome or fibromyalgia is like, the patient will often say, "Have you ever had a bad case of the flu? Do you remember what the worst day of that was like? Awful, huh? Well *that's* what *I* feel like most of the time." Some people feel like that *all* of the time!

You may experience remissions sometimes. These are the times I actually dread and hate the most. It's during this time you begin to doubt yourself. You may feel that you are "cured" or that you were never really sick in the first place. You feel well and begin to act accordingly. You overdo, in effect, thumbing your nose at The Thief. Then you experience payback. Symptoms return and your physical and emotional health suffers once again.

These symptoms are often associated with chronic fatigue syndrome and fibromyalgia. They are not in any particular order of either frequency or severity.

1. Pain between the shoulder blades

2. Head/neck ache

3. Low back pain

4. TMJ (temporomandibular joint pain)

5. Knee cap pain

6. Plantar fasciitis (pain in the soles of the feet)

7. Achilles tendonitis

8. Tennis elbow

9. Growing pains

10. Non-cardiac chest pain

11. Painful lymph nodes

12. Mitral Valve Prolapse (MVP or heart murmur). It is important to remember that if MVP is present, the patient's dentist should be made aware of this condition. A prophylactic antibiotic is often prescribed before and after any dental work is performed to help prevent infection.

13. Fatigue — not simple tiredness, but overwhelming, unable-to-move, body-and-brain-draining fatigue, to the point that if your home was on fire you could not move to safety by yourself.

14. Low-grade fever

15. Subnormal body temperature

16. Sleep disorders — either insomnia (no sleep) or hypersomnia (too much sleep). Hypersomnia, although frequent and long lasting, is non-restorative sleep.

17. Difficulty concentrating

18. Occasional confusion

19. Feeling as though you are moving about in a fog

20. Secondary depression — it's important to note that the depression experienced with The Thief is considered secondary, meaning that it's not a primary condition, but rather a result of the illness. In primary depression, patients experience symptoms such as sleep disturbances occurring during the REM stage of sleep, fatigue, loss of motivation, loss of interest in activities, apathy, feeling as if having always been depressed, can't remember *ever* having been happy, loss of hope, and suicidal thoughts or attempts at suicide. Many cases of primary depression can be successfully treated with psychological counseling and medication. In secondary depression, patients may experience symptoms such as sleep disturbances occurring during the non-REM stage of sleep, *profound* fatigue, intense frustration over being unable to do what they want to do, an awareness of not feeling as well as they used to, and hopes of feeling better. Medication is often helpful in treating secondary depression.

21. Headaches, often described as different from the usual headache

22. Chronic sore throat

23. Sudden anxiety or panic attacks

24. Severe muscle weakness

25. Worsening of PMS symptoms

26. Stiffness/gelling of the muscles

27. Visual blurring

28. Frequent urination (irritable bladder)

29. Nausea, intolerance of strong odors

30. Dizziness/vertigo

31. Muscle aches, with weakness and tenderness to touch. Pain is occasionally migratory.

32. Rapid heart rate (tachycardia)

33. Burning or prickling sensations in the face and/or extremities

34. Dry eyes

35. Dry mouth

36. Diarrhea

37. Anorexia

38. Cough

39. Morning stiffness

40. Memory impairment, especially short-term memory

41. Cognitive difficulties, which may include trouble with concentration, difficulty with organization of ideas, writing, spelling (even your own name), and difficulty with numbers

42. Irritable bowel (constipation or diarrhea or both)

43. Chronic headaches; migraines

44. Tingling and numbness in the extremities

45. Muscle twitching

46. Skin sensitivities

47. Developing allergic symptoms to food and environment

48. Heel or arch pain

49. Brain fatigue

50. Painful periods (dysmenorrhea)

51. Emotional changes: irritability, emotional lability, anxiety/panic attacks
52. Multiple chemical sensitivities
53. Joint hyper-mobility
54. Thoughts of suicide
55. Personality changes
56. Mood swings
57. Feeling unbalanced, clumsy
58. Intolerance of bright light (artificial or natural)
59. Intolerance of loud sounds
60. Low frequency sensorineural hearing loss
61. Ringing in the ears (tinnitus)
62. Exaggerated, involuntary rapid eye movement (nystagmus)
63. Vision changes: floaters, blurring, decreased depth perception, and decreased peripheral vision
64. Alcohol intolerance
65. Medication side effects increased
66. Intolerance of previously tolerated medications
67. Severe nasal and other allergies, sometimes leading to recurring sinus infections
68. Weight gain (as much as 50 pounds) or weight loss
69. Joint aches
70. Night sweats
71. Heart palpitations
72. Muscle spasms
73. Raynaud's-like symptoms
74. Carpal tunnel syndrome
75. Heartburn

76. Difficulty swallowing
77. Interstitial cystitis
78. Vivid dreams/nightmares
79. Frequent flu-like symptoms
80. Carbohydrate cravings
81. Difficulty breathing with exertion
82. Reduced libido
83. Swelling of fingers
84. Slight speech impairment
85. Restless legs
86. Pain during intercourse

It should be understood that many of these symptoms are also found in other chronic illnesses. Most likely, you will not experience *all* of these symptoms. Chances are you will experience different symptoms at different times. They may be constant or they may wax and wane. New

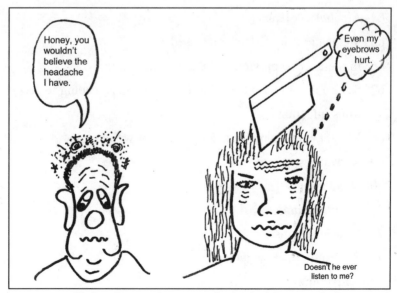

Oh, how I want to hurt you....if only I had the strength.

symptoms may develop at any time. There is simply no way to predict how any one person will be affected. That's why it's important to remember that when someone says they're sick or in pain — *believe them.* It's bad enough to be suffering, but it's worse when you're not believed.

Here's a story about Sophia that shows how much relief she felt when she was finally believed by others in her life.

SOPHIA

Sophia was a stay-at-home mom. She never knew her capabilities, her strengths. Indeed, she never knew she had either.

When her "fledgling" left the nest, Sophia began to spread her own wings, deciding she wanted to see if she could make it in college. It had been twenty years since she last attended school and she was afraid she might fail. But her newfound adventurous spirit took over and Sophia embarked upon a journey of self-discovery. She learned to her delight that she was capable, she was intelligent. She had something to offer. It never ceased to amaze her when people sought her out for her opinion. She felt — important.

Sophia reveled in her new role. Life was good. For a while. Then suddenly her life was in turmoil. Everyone who was near and dear to her — her husband, child, mother, and even she, herself, each suffered serious and, in some cases, life-threatening illnesses.

Her mother succumbed to breast cancer. Sophia felt that she should be the one to deal with all the details of her mother's death. Even though she had younger siblings who would have gladly helped, Sophia felt deeply that she had to protect them. She loved them fiercely and wanted to shield them, to spare them from the pain that she was feeling. She didn't want them to hurt as she did.

When Sophia was cleaning out her mom's apartment, she decided to start with the bathroom. The bathroom is such a personal place and would be the most difficult to deal with. The first thing she saw when she began packing was her mom's breast prosthesis. That nearly did her in, but she managed to keep her resolve. Thank God her siblings didn't find it, she thought. Finding such a personal part of their mother would have devastated them and that would have destroyed Sophia. What would she or could she say to them?

Sophia did such a good job holding it together that she didn't even cry at her mother's funeral. In fact, it was two months before the tears began to fall. She thought herself a monster for being unable to express her sadness. She loved and missed her mother. Why couldn't she cry?

When a good friend heard about Sophia's inability to cry for her mom and for herself, she brought her a magazine article about a family that had just lost their mom. That did it! Her friend had given her what she needed so desperately — the gift of tears. Sophia could no longer hold it in. The walls came tumbling down and down until Sophia felt like a limp rag. Now she felt she could live again.

After much thought Sophia left a job she loved and was good at. She left behind many good friends. She moved to another state, to a new home that she was in the process of building. She found her dream job, but the dream turned into a nightmare. The stress was unimaginable. After a time common sense took over, she gave her notice, and left the job and the stress behind.

But she traded that stress for another, because now that she was out of work, she was also without health insurance and had to depend on her husband's coverage. This forced her to travel over 75 miles each time she needed to see her doctor, which was becoming quite frequent because she was just not feeling right. She was in pain, wasn't sleeping at all, and was forgetting things — to the point that she thought she had the beginning signs of Alzheimer's. She had irritable bowel, and those headaches! She had always had headaches, but these were different. She couldn't explain how they were different. They were just different.

Before long, her days were spent lying on the couch with the television on and her back to it. Maybe those doctors and some of her friends were right. Maybe it was all in her head. Maybe she was a lazy hypochondriac. It didn't occur to her that she was depressed. Her husband was about the only one who really believed her.

Finally, one of the many doctors she had seen said to her, "You have fibromyalgia. Here's a pamphlet. You have one more visit left on your insurance referral and that's the last I'll see of you." Then he left the room.

Her life began again that day, and as she read the pamphlet, Sophia's depression lifted almost visibly. She smiled as she learned she had an incurable illness. Incurable, but at least she finally knew what it was. It had a name and other people had it, too. She wasn't alone anymore! Finally there were some answers to her questions.

She found herself wanting to know more about her illness. She read anything and everything she could get her hands on. She was still bothered by her many symptoms, but she learned to cope with them.

Then she heard about a support group that met during the day. Well, that's okay, she didn't work anymore and her symptoms had progressed to the point she couldn't work anymore. She decided to give the support group a try. Hesitantly, she wandered in to the meeting and was amazed at the number of people there. Sophia was welcomed with open arms. She couldn't believe it! "All these people and they have the same illness I do! They know how I feel. They believe me." Her head swam with all the information she was taking in and the meeting was over way too fast.

Sophia barely made it to her car before she burst into tears. She felt she had just become a member of a special family. It wasn't long before she teamed up with Lauren and Helen and the three of them started a support group in another city. Life was livable once again.

4
WHO GETS IT AND WHAT IS IT LIKE?

Life is one long process of getting tired.
— Samuel Butler

Butcher, baker, candlestick maker, doctor, lawyer, Indian chief. No one is immune to this equal opportunity, non-discriminatory illness. Race, age, and religion make no difference to The Thief. This illness affects you financially, socially, physically, emotionally, and sexually. Chances are if you don't have the illness yourself, you know someone who does.

Imagine that every person who has CFS or FM has at least two people in their life, such as a spouse and child. That means there are literally millions of people *affected* by these illnesses.

Women are more likely to be diagnosed with CFS or fibromyalgia. No one knows why. It may be that women are more aware of their bodies and know when something is wrong.

Traditionally, women are the nurturers and caregivers. They care for the children and the husband. They tend the home and keep things running smoothly. Many also work outside of the home. Women *need* to be well, so are more likely to seek a doctor's care when they feel something is wrong. It also seems that women are more interested in finding out *why* they feel what they feel. And it may be that women are more sensitive to pain and emotions than men. As a rule, men are encouraged or expected to accept pain, as complaining may be seen as a sign of weakness, and most men don't want to be viewed as weak.

Perhaps the most heart-wrenching victims of this illness are the children — the ones who have the illness and the ones who love someone who is afflicted.

That's right — age is not a factor when it comes to CFS. Children's complaints are often dismissed as "growing pains." They are given a pat on the head, a glass of milk, and a cookie, and told to go out and play.

What is wrong with this response? **IT DOESN'T HURT TO GROW!** There is no such thing as growing pains.

Children want to go to school and play with their friends. Listen, and believe children when they tell you they don't feel well and then do something to let them know you believe them. Don't doubt them. Investigate to get to the root of the problem.

Parents, children, and medical professionals are often unaware of the existence, manifestations, and severity of CFS symptoms in children. Because of the unpredictability of their symptoms and the reluctance to believe that children can, and do, get this illness, there are very few statistics about the frequency of chronic fatigue syndrome in children. However, some studies done in Britain have found that *"this illness is responsible for forty-two percent"* of all long-term school absences. The children afflicted are often inaccurately labeled with behavior problems, school-phobia, or depression. Parents are often accused of encouraging this behavior and often the sick child and the family are subjected to the trauma of being dragged through the court and social services because of this erroneous belief. The school phobic is well when allowed to stay home. The child who is a victim of CFS is sick all weekend from trying to cope during the week's school routine.

From newborn baby to grandparent, everyone must meet and master certain developmental milestones before moving on to the next. The toddler learns to eat and walk on his own and be less dependent on mom. The young adult learns to develop relationships outside of and separate from his family before he can move on to starting and nurturing a family of his own. A chronic illness often delays the mastering of these important milestones, thereby delaying psychological and psychosocial maturation.

Obviously, children do not like being different from their peers. They do not like being labeled as sick. They prefer to be with other children, doing what other children do: going to school, playing, learning, and being naturally active. Healthy children are able to achieve this "normalcy." Children with chronic fatigue syndrome find normalcy difficult.

This illness does *not* present as a psychological or motivational problem in children or adults. Indeed, it is *not* a psychological or motivational problem. Children are motivated! Children with CFS simply can't perform at the same level as others their age due to the physical, cognitive, and neurological symptoms they experience.

But it's not impossible for the child with CFS to gain an education. A lot of accommodation, planning, and flexibility is necessary, but it can and must be done. Some students with CFS have finished high school and gone to their own graduation. Some have graduated with the rest of their class while never setting foot inside of a classroom or attending the graduation ceremony. Some have gone on to complete college. These young people are to be admired and held up as an inspiration. They have persevered and shown that while they are weak, they are also strong. They have overcome what life has thrown at them and shown inner strength and ingenuity in meeting those challenges.

For more information about chronic fatigue syndrome in children and how to help them, their families, and school officials, you can order "Guidelines for Children with CFIDS" from the National CFIDS Foundation, 103 Aletha Road, Needham, MA 02492-3931, Phone: 781-449-3535.

WHAT CAUSES IT?

Before you can treat or cure an illness, whether it's acute or chronic, you must know how it is acquired. There are many ways to acquire an illness. It may be contagious — one that someone you have been in contact with has passed on to you. Or it may be a familial illness, one that is passed on genetically within a family. It may be an illness that occurs within specific racial groups, for example, Tay-Sachs disease or sickle-cell anemia.

So what category does CFS fall in? A few years ago it was anybody's guess, but in 2006, scientists found that a virus may be the cause of CFS. The press release that contained this exciting news brought new hope to us all. We felt validated. It isn't all in our heads! We have an *illness* and *not* a syndrome, or a bunch of symptoms grouped together.

While these researchers still believe that a virus may cause CFS, it hasn't yet been proven and more work must be done. Our hopes have been raised and dashed before in the search for the cause, which must come before a cure can be developed. But I am assured that researchers are very, very close. Research being done on many fronts is beginning to dovetail and results are being proven and replicated. Tests are being developed. It won't be long before we can say, "We found the cause, now let's find the cure."

Most of the research is focusing on a virus being the cause of CFS, and that makes a lot of sense when you understand how viruses work. Since viruses are contagious, CFS is also potentially contagious. There are still no definitive tests or treatment that will work for everyone and it is still, at this time, incurable. The treatment remains the same: managing symptoms by reducing pain and improving sleep.

Now for the million-dollar question — what is a virus? A virus is a tiny organism, about one-millionth of an inch and one thousand times smaller than bacteria. They are so small they can only be seen with an electron microscope. Viruses differ from bacteria in that bacteria are living organisms that act the same way other living organisms do: they absorb nutrients, grow, and reproduce. They do not need any chemical reactions to live and they reproduce by cell division.

A virus is more like a parasite in that it cannot function without a host. It attaches itself to the host cell in order to survive and reproduce. When a virus enters a host cell, it takes over and starts issuing new instructions to the cell using that cell's enzymes to accomplish its goal. Soon, new copies of the virus are being produced.

A virus can't stay in the host cell forever, so when it's time to leave, it does so by one of two ways, either by breaking through the cell's membrane thereby destroying that cell, or by breaking out and attaching to the outer surface of the cell. Once the virus leaves the cell it rapidly attacks other cells, reproducing quickly and spreading throughout the body.

How do viruses enter your body? Through the air you breathe when someone coughs or sneezes, by contact with body fluids, or through a break in the skin. Once a virus gains entry to the body all it needs is a host cell.

Some viruses do not replicate immediately. They enter the host cell and mix their instructions with the host cell's instructions and become dormant until "awakened" and called into action. Depending on the virus, this dormant period may last for years. Once awakened, the virus's genetic instructions take over the host cell and begin to reproduce. No one knows exactly what determines just when a virus will awaken. The reasons could be environmental or it could be pre-programmed, like an alarm clock. It could even possibly be stress that awakens the sleeping virus. So you see how it is possible for a virus to live in its host for years while the person carrying it is unaware, because he has no symptoms.

Your body is an amazing machine, capable of repairing itself, in most cases on the job 24/7/365, striving to maintain optimal health. Yet, for years many sick people have believed that all they need to cure what ails them is a pill. They are unwilling to let nature take its course, hence the old saying, "Treat a cold it lasts a week, don't treat it and it lasts seven days."

The demand for "a pill" to cure all our ills is the reason some antibiotics are no longer effective. Many people do not understand that antibiotics are not effective in treating viruses, because anything that will kill a virus will also kill its host cell. That's why vaccines were developed.

For some viral diseases, immunization works by injecting a small amount of a virus into the body in order to produce an antigen so the body will produce antibodies that it can recognize if the virus enters your body again. If that virus should enter your body again, your antibodies

VIRUS	BACTERIA
Size: one-millionth of an inch	Size: one micrometer (1,000 times larger than a virus)
Needs a host cell in order to function	Can function (eat, reproduce) independently
Can remain dormant in a host cell for years without producing symptoms	Does not have a long life span
Antibiotics ineffective; vaccines helpful	Antibiotics are effective, some vaccines also
Is never beneficial	Some bacteria can be helpful and are needed by the body. For example, bacteria found in the intestines.

will search out the antigens, attach themselves to it, and then kill and dispose of the virus.

Madge's story underscores how the uncertainty about how our illness is acquired can affect a person's physical and emotional health.

MADGE

Madge is a busy, sensible, outgoing, take-no-prisoners type of woman. You can't get away with much of anything where she's concerned. Not for long anyway. Her kids know that from long experience.

When you have a large family, as Madge does, (including a large extended family of relatives and friends, and kids' friends) you don't have the time, patience, or energy to do anything but get to the nitty-gritty right away. Everyone in that family — and extended family — works hard and plays hard. They fight amongst themselves, but close ranks and turn as one against any threat against one of their own.

Madge is a matriarch who loves and protects her family unreservedly. She gives wise, loving, and truthful counsel. Each child (and sometimes her children's friends) seeks her advice and help with their problems. Madge somehow manages to make each child feel as if that one is her favorite.

Madge had no problem adjusting to her empty nest when all of her "chicks" flew the coop. In fact, she reveled in it. She was having a high old time of it. Finally it was her turn.

The only problem was she was beginning to have some health problems. Not fatal ones, but definitely painful ones. She wondered if she had always had the pain but was too busy to notice. No, she didn't think so. Being an intelligent and curious woman, Madge began researching her symptoms. She went to doctor after doctor and it took some time to finally settle on a medical routine that helped. But just as she was getting comfortable in that routine, some of her adult children began to exhibit similar, troubling symptoms. Her heart was filled with dread. Had she passed her health problems on to her children? Yeah, it looks as if she might have.

A mother is a strong person. She can handle most anything life throws at her. But when her children are suffering — and she thinks she's the cause — and she can't take away their pain — well, that is a special kind of hell. Madge finds it difficult enough to handle her own pain, but believing that she may have passed her painful condition on to her beloved children and grandchildren is a source of extreme and constant stress to her. And since stress leads to worsening symptoms, Madge's pain, both physical and emotional, has reached an almost unbearable level. Intellectually, she knows she has no control over her genetic legacy. But her heart rules her head and she finds it difficult to accept. She feels her children's pain as keenly as she feels her own.

Madge loves research, so she is always bringing new information to her other support group members and sharing information with her children as well (even those in denial). Other members of her group will also bring in copies of articles to share, and, when they do, they bring extras for Madge to give to her family. Madge's pain is double or triple anyone else's because she also has a couple of other painful conditions, and because she may have passed her illness on to her children.

Madge's most valuable contribution is her ability to see three sides to a problem that seems to have only two sides. She loves playing the devil's advocate and does so frequently. Her questions (and answers) are informed, well thought out, and incisive. By collecting and sharing information, Madge feels she's doing something positive and necessary to help her family and others who suffer from CFS.

HEALTH AND HYGIENE 101

Let's examine how you can help prevent a virus from entering your body. Your body's defenses are constantly at work trying to maintain optimal health. As soon as a virus enters your body, your immune system kicks in and gets to work. Pyrogens are produced, causing you to get a fever. Heat slows down the virus and inhibits its ability to reproduce. This reaction of the immune system continues until the virus is eliminated. With your immune system doing all it can, it's up to you to help it along by using simple, common-sense precautions to reduce the chance of spreading germs:

- Cover your mouth when coughing or sneezing; use disposable tissues instead of cloth handkerchiefs.

- Avoid contact with the body fluids of others.

- Wash your hands frequently with soap for a minimum of one minute.

- Avoid contact with those who are sick and showing symptoms.

- Drink lots of fluids, get plenty of rest, eat a proper diet, and contact your physician if symptoms persist or worsen.

- If you are sick, stay home from school or work. No one wants your germs, so don't spread them around. Especially avoid contact with infants, the elderly, and people on chemotherapy, as these groups do not have strong immune systems and germs are very opportunistic.

- Remember, a temperature of up to 102°F is helping to fight the illness, but you need to seek medical attention if your temperature goes higher, or persists for several days.

AS THE DISEASE PROGRESSES

CFS and fibromyalgia are difficult illnesses to diagnose, treat, and understand. They are fraught with definite ifs and maybes. The symptoms are similar, almost to the point of being one illness, but they react differently with each person who has either illness. For example, suppose there are only ten diagnostic symptoms. I could suffer from symptoms 1, 3, 6, 7, and 10. I can now be diagnosed with the illness. However, you could suffer from symptoms 2, 4, 6, 8, and 10 and you would be diagnosed with the same illness. Two people with different symptoms yet diagnosed with the same illness. Now, throw in the factor that it is possible to have CFS without having fibromyalgia and vice-versa, and it is also possible to have *both* CFS and fibromyalgia. Are you confused yet?

The course and prognosis of the disease cannot be predicted either. One person may experience a very slow onset and have mild symptoms. Another may have a rapid onset and become bedridden. Some people may have a slow onset and continue to develop symptoms that are mild at first and later become serious. I believe the difficulty in plotting the course and progression of CFS may be due to the cause of CFS. If it is caused by a virus, it is not like the common cold virus. You know what course a cold will take and that you will eventually recover.

You may be particularly nice to yourself and keep in shape, but when your CFS becomes active and you experience a flare, there's precious little you can do to stop it. Usually the flare will subside and you will feel well again, but that's not guaranteed, because your body can't seem to get rid of it.

Flares are inevitable. Take good care of yourself, don't fight them, and learn to adjust your life according to your illness. Fighting flares uses valuable energy that you cannot afford. You'll get over a flare faster if you don't fight it at all.

REMISSIONS

When you're feeling good you feel almost invincible. This is called a remission. I must confess that as much as I hate this illness, I hate the remissions almost as much, because I begin to feel that the doctors and I were wrong, that I'm not sick, it must have been something else, and I'm now cured! WHOOOOPEEE!!! I begin to act accordingly. I'm super-woman once again, doing all I can to make up for lost time. And then, inevitably, it happens again — a flare of symptoms reminds me who the real boss is. But, to my credit, I am learning. I do things in moderation now, even though I'm tempted to overdo. I've learned to plan, organize my life, *and* I have learned to say "no" without feeling guilty.

A valued member of our support group has what she calls the "fifty percent rule." What is the 50%? Well, if you plan to walk a mile — walk only a half mile instead. Do only 50% of what you wanted or planned to do. As Lisa puts it, "Don't overbook the flight."

When you're feeling good, you will be tempted to plan a full week-end of activities with family and friends. But, I can almost guarantee that if you do, you will end up in bed and the fun weekend will have to be canceled — for you at least. Be sensible. If you have a full, active day planned one day, then *plan* on spending the next day in bed. Include some necessary down time in your plans, so you don't end up disappointing yourself and others by having to cancel. Plan smart. Be smart.

WHAT BRINGS ON A FLARE AND WHAT CAN YOU DO ?

Certain physical, emotional, and environmental factors can aggravate symptoms that are already present or work to trigger a flare if you are in remission. Here are some of the most important ones.

1. **Stress.** Stress is stress, whether it's good (winning the lottery) or bad (the death of a loved one). Your body can't differentiate between good and bad stress — it can only react.

2. **Being especially active (overdoing).** Perhaps you were feeling good, so you exercised a little too strenuously, or you went out and raked the yard, then came in and rearranged the living room after shampooing the rug. Forget your thoughts of recrimination. Fill the tub with comfortably warm water and soak for as long as you like. Have a light meal, take your pain medication, and go to bed. Other treatments that work for some: ask your partner for a massage, practice relaxation techniques, apply moist heat or cold packs to the affected areas, practice Reiki, try meditation, get involved in something you are really interested in, read a good book (or a bad book — that may make you fall asleep faster).

3. **Drafts**, such as from open doors, fans, and air conditioners. If you can't tolerate lower temperatures and your family can't tolerate the heat and lack of air circulation, stay away from that open door or air conditioner, wear layers of clothing, and try to reach an agreement with the rest of the family as to how low they can go on the thermostat and how high you can go. Try to find a comfortable temperature for all.

4. **Weather changes** such as barometric pressure, dampness, and humidity. There is little you can do about changes in the weather except to expect them and be prepared for them. Know how they affect you and plan accordingly. Some people can sense changes in barometric pressure because they get migraines, or because their mood changes, or because their pain level increases. This is a personal call, so figure out what works for you. During those

lazy, hazy days of summer when it's hot and the air is so dense you can cut it with a knife, dress in layers of light clothing, use a dehumidifier, and keep your activities to the barest minimum.

5. **Loud noises and bright lights.** These have a devastating affect on me. I am bombarded with unpleasant sensory input that builds to the point of actual physical pain, and, at times, anxiety attack. If you experience this too, you need to explain this fact to friends and family. They will try to understand and be sympathetic to your needs. I remember an incident at my sister-in-law's home during a holiday get-together. Outside an icy rain fell. Inside there were over thirty people, about one-third of them children under the age of ten. Of course everyone was excited and talking at once, and every light in the house was on. I did what I could to escape from this sensory overload. I went upstairs, I hid in a closet, I even went outside for a while, but nothing was working and I became more and more anxious, nearing a panic attack. I couldn't believe it when I found myself standing up and YELLING, "Quiet down! Please!" I totally embarrassed myself. But, they were my family and they proved they loved me by inviting me back the next year.

6. **Being too hot or too cold.** This needs little explanation. Dress in layers and seek a comfortable temperature.

7. Staying in one position for a prolonged period of time, such as during a long car trip or attending a lengthy movie or concert. Stop the car and get out, walk around a bit to stretch your arms and legs, twist and turn to work out the kinks. In a building you can do the same thing (quietly). Excuse yourself and walk to the back of the theater and stretch.

8. **Repetitive motion.** This can lead to carpal tunnel syndrome and other repetitive use injuries. Working with the arms elevated above the head especially can cause a sustained contraction of the muscles that leads to pain. If the problem is brought about in the work place, ask your supervisor if you can trade jobs with someone else or make other accommodations. It's better for everyone involved to prevent illness or injury than to have to try to correct it.

9. **Infection that stresses the body and immune system.** In addition to the earlier tips on preventing infection, you can also wipe the phone receiver with alcohol before and after use, take zinc tablets at the first sign of a cold, get flu and pneumonia vaccinations, get plenty of exercise, and see your doctor at the first sign of an infection. Don't insist on an antibiotic for minor infections.

10. **Non-restorative sleep.** Your bedroom should be used for sleep and lovemaking. It's important to develop healthy sleep hygiene. Go to bed at the same time each night and rise at the same time each morning. Leave your worries in the next room. Your bedroom should be quiet and pleasant, with no distractions and no television. Do not eat or drink just before going to bed. Avoid alcohol and caffeine late in the day. Caffeine is a stimulant; and while alcohol acts first as a sedative it acts later as a stimulant. You should invest in a comfortable mattress and pillow, and keep your room at a comfortable sleeping temperature. Finally drugs such as Benadryl or Elavil can help. If, however, these suggestions haven't helped after a few months, see your primary physician to discuss your sleep problems and explore whether a sleep study is in order.

11. **Pain.** Pain is a valuable symptom, not an expected condition. Pain tells you that something is wrong. Talk to your physician about it and keep talking (to other doctors if necessary) until you can manage your pain, or better yet, it disappears completely.

12. **Fatigue.** Prolonged, debilitating fatigue is not normal. Talk to your physician and keep talking until you find answers. For these last two symptoms you will be very lucky if the first doctor you speak to has all the right answers, but if he doesn't, look for another doctor, and keep looking until you find just the right one. Remember to keep a written record of all your doctor visits, what

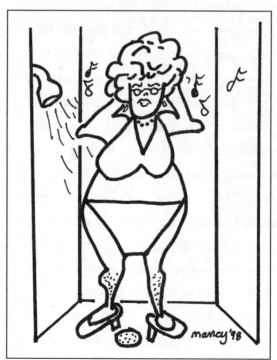

"Why do I have the feeling I've forgotten something"
Another forgettable moment courtesy of FM/CFS

they said, what they did, and how their suggestions and treatments worked out.

So, basically you handle a flare by staying calm, relaxed, and knowing that "this too shall pass." Get more sleep, even if you have to schedule it. Take more breaks in your activities. Treat yourself well. Stay clear of any type of physical or emotional stress that can act as triggers.

If holding it in gets to be too much, feel free to vent — to your spouse, friend, next-door neighbor, or your Aunt Sadie. If you're too shy to speak, write it down. Find a hobby or something pleasant to occupy your mind and help you forget your pain and worry. And, last but not least, turn your problems over to a higher power. God does not give you more than you can bear. He's there to take care of you. Ask for help; He will hear you and help you through this.

5
BODY SYSTEMS AND THE THIEF

Health is better than medicine.
— Unknown

The Thief affects its victims physically, emotionally, socially, financially, and sexually. It affects every system in the body. Please remember
that no matter what you call our illness, whether you call it fibromyalgia
or chronic fatigue syndrome, they are both considered syndromes. A
syndrome is a collection of symptoms so common that a clinical picture
is possible. What follows is a brief description of body systems and
common symptoms experienced by victims of The Thief.

INTEGUMENTARY SYSTEM
The integumentary system consists of the skin, hair, and nails. The
skin is the body's largest organ. It functions as a guardian, protecting the
body from unwanted invaders (such as bacteria) and preventing the loss
of body fluids. In addition, the skin provides you with sensations such as
touch and pain.

The Thief's effects on the integumentary system

1. Rosacea — literally means "rosy, red rash"; a form of acne usually found on the "T-zone" of the face.

2. Dry skin — especially on the face, but also in patches elsewhere on the body. The eyes, nose, mucus membranes, and vaginal area can also be affected. It's no wonder that our skin becomes dry. The average person loses between 600 cc and 900 cc of water per day through perspiration. In addition, the skin acts as a barrier, making absorption difficult. To combat dryness, avoid products that contain ingredients that further dry the skin (e.g. alcohol). In order to do this you must read labels (a theme you will hear frequently in this book), practice good hygiene, drink plenty of fluids, and decrease exposure to the sun. Don't feel you must avoid the sun altogether, however, because some sun is needed to make vitamin D. But, be aware that some medications will make the effects of the sun worse, so be careful. Be a label reader and check with your pharmacist. Eye drops, nasal spray, imitation saliva, and vaginal lubricants can also help with dryness problems.

3. Nails — become brittle, develop lines, and may become yellowish in color. Sometimes the "moon" is missing, white spots appear.

4. Hair loss — possibly due to vitamin deficiency, also seen in cases of low thyroid function (hypothyroidism). Receding hairline is possible, sometimes with loss of hair on legs/arms also.

5. Sun sensitivity — resulting in rashes, hives, and eye pain from the brightness. Using sun block (the higher the number the bet-

ter) and reapplying frequently will help, as well as wearing a wide-brimmed hat and extra dark sunglasses.

6. Raynaud's phenomenon — this is a vascular condition that is the result of an underlying disease and not the primary disease. The tips of fingers and toes (and sometimes ears and tip of nose) feel painfully, icy cold, and a change in skin color (blue to white) of the affected areas is noted.

THE RESPIRATORY SYSTEM

The respiratory system consists of the mouth, nose, throat, lungs, and chest wall along with their associated structures. The respiratory system's function is to take oxygen from the air you breathe and transfer it to your blood, and to take waste product (carbon dioxide) from your blood and transfer it to the air.

The Thief's effects on the respiratory system

1. Sore throat — warm salt-water gargles provide some temporary relief, however, if accompanied by a fever, or your throat is red, or has white patches, see your doctor.

2. Non-cardiac chest pain — usually referred to as chest wall pain, is not cardiac in origin, although it may feel like it.

3. Painful lymph nodes

4. Pulmonary (lung) infections — because your immune system is not working at peak efficiency, you are susceptible to opportunistic bacterial, fungal, or yeast infections.

5. Shortness of breath/heaviness in the chest — can be caused by low blood volume or due to overworking yourself after a period of exhaustion.

THE CIRCULATORY SYSTEM

The circulatory system consists of the heart and blood and lymph vessels. The circulatory system functions in delivery and removal also. It delivers products (such as oxygen) vital to the normal functioning of the body's cells, organs, and glands, and then it removes some of the body's wastes.

The Thief's effects on the circulatory system

1. Raynaud's phenomenon — off and on attacks of ischemia (decreased blood flow) to the tips of the extremities (fingertips, toes, nose), Raynaud's is a painful condition brought on by cold or stress. It is usually treated with medication, decreasing stress, and applying heat to affected areas.

2. Mitral valve prolapse (MVP) — or heart murmur, often a benign condition, usually requiring no treatment. It may be caused by an especially active trigger point. Antibiotic prophylaxis before and after dental work may be required if you have MVP. Make sure your dentist is aware of your condition.

3. Headaches/migraines — Constriction of blood vessels to the brain causing pain, sometimes severe. Can be triggered by certain foods, stress, or changes in weather. Drug treatment varies from analgesics to ergotamines or anti-hypertensives. Some patients find that a cool/cold, dark, quiet room with no distractions can be helpful.

4. Lightheadedness — possibly caused by lack of restorative sleep or poor circulation to the head because of low blood perfusion.

5. Low blood perfusion (low blood volume) — for some reason the volume of blood in a person with chronic fatigue syndrome (PWC) is lower than that of a healthy person. The blood is also

thicker, making circulation slow and "sludgy," sort of like the oil in a car that has never had an oil change. That fact, combined with the poor sleep patterns of the PWC may be the cause of many of the symptoms found in our illness, including cognitive difficulties, memory problems, and impaired coordination.

6. Orthostatic hypotension (sudden drop in blood pressure when a person stands up after sitting or lying down) — This may cause symptoms ranging from dizziness to headaches and anything in between.

THE GASTROINTESTINAL SYSTEM

The gastrointestinal system consists of the mouth, tongue, teeth, throat, esophagus, stomach, large and small intestines, liver, pancreas, and gall bladder. The gastrointestinal system ingests, digests, and absorbs nutrients from food products, and eliminates indigestible waste.

The Thief's effects on the GI system:

1. Irritable bowel — abdominal pain often accompanied by alternating bouts of constipation and diarrhea. Symptoms often occur without warning and can be treated with psychotherapy, biofeedback, certain medications, and a diet high in bran and fiber.

2. Celiac disease — This is an illness of impaired absorption and hypersensitivity to cereal grains and gluten. This illness could rapidly lead to dehydration. It is important to become a label reader if you have this disease, because you need to be on a gluten-free diet.

3. Swollen glands

4. Tooth decay — possibly caused by dry mouth.

5. Yeast infections — though a naturally occurring organism in the body, the opportunistic overgrowth of yeast can wreak havoc on those with a compromised immune system, such as those with The Thief. A yeast infection often gets its start from the use/overuse of antibiotics, eating too much sugar, or from a diet high in carbohydrates. Treatment usually consists of restricting carbohydrate intake, reducing sugar intake, and an antifungal medication. Personally, I find that acidophilus (a bacteria found in yogurt and other places that promotes intestinal health) works great for me, but I suggest you do as I did, and talk it over with your doctor first.

6. Abdominal pain — may arise from many causes including poor diet and irritable bowel syndrome.

7. Bloating

8. Heartburn — which, by the way, has nothing to do with your heart. Heartburn occurs when the contents of the stomach back up into the esophagus. If this occurs frequently enough, it will cause the esophagus to erode. Antacids will help temporarily, but you should see your physician and change your diet, avoiding foods that bring on heartburn.

9. Dry mouth — a common problem for people with chronic fatigue syndrome or fibromyalgia. Drink extra fluids or use imitation saliva. A dry mouth can lead to tooth decay.

THE URINARY SYSTEM

The urinary system consists of the kidneys, ureters, bladder, and urethra. Its function is the formation and excretion of the waste product urine.

The Thief's effects on the urinary system:

1. Urinary frequency — may be caused by always feeling "dry" which results in drinking extra fluids to replace what we lose.

2. Frequent urinary tract infections (UTI) — may be caused by poor hygiene or not drinking enough fluids. The vaginal area is a perfect environment for the growth of bacteria because bacteria like a warm, dark, moist area to grow. Diagnosis is usually made by performing a urine culture to confirm the presence of infection, followed by antibiotic treatment. Meanwhile, increase fluid intake, (cranberry juice and vitamin C can also help because they create an acid environment that bacteria don't like), "peri" wash/rinse after urinating, and never put off urinating when you need to or hold it in. When you have to "go" — just go!

3. Painful urination — see your doctor to determine the cause.

THE ENDOCRINE SYSTEM AND REPRODUCTIVE SYSTEM

These two systems work together and are linked in the female by the ovaries. In the female, the reproductive system consists of the ovaries, fallopian tubes, uterus, and the vagina. In the male, the reproductive system consists of the testes, scrotum, penis, urethra, and vas deferens The function of the reproductive system is the continuation of the species and bonding.

The endocrine system consists of the pituitary gland, thyroid, parathyroid, adrenal glands, pancreas, ovaries (or testes in males), and thymus gland. The endocrine system produces and secretes hormones that affect many body systems and functions.

The Thief's effects on the endocrine and reproductive systems:

1. Hypothyroidism, hyperthyroidism — the thyroid gland is responsible for secreting hormones necessary for growth and metabolism, and also as a storehouse for iodine. Hypothyroidism is caused by a thyroid gland that is not functioning or barely functioning. A person with hypothyroidism is lethargic, drowsy, fatigued, and gains weight. A person with hyperthyroidism produces excessive thyroid hormones, which causes the opposite effect. These people are generally "balls of fire," always on the go, tend to be skinny, have a fast heart rate, and are restless insomniacs. See your doctor for treatment of either of these conditions.

2. Reaction to stress — more on this later.

3. Painful menses (dysmenorrhea) — there are many possible reasons for this problem and you should see your doctor to establish the cause. Apply heat to the affected area, get lots of rest, wear loose fitting clothing, and avoid constipation.

4. Painful intercourse (dyspareunia) — the cause may be as simple as vaginal dryness, but could be something more serious. Consult with your doctor to find the cause and determine treatment.

5. Regulation of menses — see your doctor.

6. Painful ovulation — see your doctor.

7. Endometriosis — an overgrowth of endometrial tissue, often causing excessive menstrual bleeding, pelvic pain/pressure, and fertility problems. See your doctor for diagnosis and treatment.

8. Difficulty conceiving — see your doctor.

THE NERVOUS SYSTEM

The nervous system is extremely complex and consists of the central nervous system and the peripheral nervous system. The brain, spinal cord, and nerves are part of the central nervous system. The peripheral nervous system consists of the nerves and ganglia outside of the brain and spinal cord. The function of the nervous system is to communicate and coordinate information and instructions from the brain to the body and the body to the brain.

The Thief's effects on the nervous system:

1. Fluctuation of brain chemistry — causing loss of sleep, forgetfulness, feeling as if you are in a fog, lightheadedness, and dizziness.

2. Hyper-reaction to, and recognition of, pain or painful stimuli.

3. Sensitivity to bright light, either artificial or natural — I know this one well. When confronted with bright lights I feel as if I am being bombarded with obnoxious stimuli, causing me actual physical pain. I have been known to wear two pair of sunglasses when the sun is extra bright or reflecting off the snow.

4. Sensitivity to loud sounds — As with bright lights, it's almost as if the internal switch that enables your body to "shut off" the stimuli is broken or miswired.

5. Sensitivity to strong odors — Strong odors cause headaches and nausea in many people.

6. Headaches/migraines.

7. "Fibro-fog" — confusion and forgetfulness.

8. Sleep disturbance — Sleep is required for your body to repair itself. When you are deprived of restorative sleep, your body cannot heal and each problem you have intensifies with lack of

sleep. If you were to intentionally deny yourself sleep for three days, you would begin to experience symptoms such as fatigue, irritability, and poor coordination. In other words, symptoms the people with chronic fatigue syndrome experience daily. Practice good sleep hygiene. Go to bed at the same time; get up at the same time, and don't allow television or other distractions in the bedroom. A sleep study could prove invaluable in helping determine just what your sleep problem is so you and your doctor can work on getting you a good, restful night's sleep.

9. Activation of fight-or-flight response (panic attacks) — the immune system is depressed; the adrenals cause the heart to beat faster and metabolism to increase. See more in chapter on stress.

10. Secondary depression — this would be depression that is a result of the illness. It is not the same as primary depression, which is an illness in itself.

11. Cognitive difficulties — difficulty dealing with numbers and words. Some people even have difficulty spelling their own name.

12. Memory problems — especially short-term memory.

13. Impaired coordination.

14. Dizziness/lightheadedness.

15. Vertigo — not the same as dizziness. Dizziness is a sensation. Vertigo is the result of a disease or condition that elicits the sensation of dizziness.

THE MUSCULOSKELETAL SYSTEM

The musculoskeletal system consists of bones, muscles, joints, cartilage, ligaments, tendons, and bursas. The musculoskeletal system supports your body, allows it to move, and protects all internal structures.

There are 206 bones in the human body. Each bone is connected by joints. Each joint is covered by connective tissue (cartilage), and there are literally hundreds of muscles in the body.

This is where The Thief does most of his dirty work, and the name FIBROMYALGIA says it all. When the word fibromyalgia is broken down, the illness is well described:

"fibro" — refers to the fibrous tissues of the body (tendons, ligaments)

"my" — refers to the muscles (I know you feel as if the pain is in the bone, but it's not. It's in the muscles.)

"algia" — means pain

So literally, fibromyalgia means pain in the muscles and the tissues that surround them.

When a muscle contracts, you feel the muscle tighten, and this can sometimes be painful. Consider now the location of some of those muscles and you will understand the reason for your pain. The uterus is a muscle, as is the colon (abdominal pain). The muscles of the back (especially between the shoulders), the temporomandibular joint (TMJ) (the temples and the jaw), and the head (headaches) are also areas that often cause problems for fibromyalgia patients.

The Thief's effects on the musculoskeletal system:

1. Pain — muscle pain.
2. Kneecap pain.

3. Plantar fasciitis — heel pain, which can be excruciating. (Think about it. Those few, small bones support the entire weight of your body. Is it any wonder we get foot pain?)

4. Back pain.

5. Carpal tunnel syndrome — repetitive movement disorder.

6. Temporomandibular joint (TMJ) — results in jaw pain.

7. Leg pain.

8. Hip pain.

9. Elbow pain.

Knowing the definition of the word fibromyalgia helps you understand the reason for your pain. Treat your symptoms as they occur. Use common sense. Practice good posture. If the symptoms become overwhelming and you don't know which to treat first, treat the "fire of the moment." Treat the worst problem and get that under control. Don't try to fix everything at once.

Chances are this has happened to you before. You're experienced now. Do what you need to do. Will a warm bath help? How about a long nap? Or medication? Reiki? Meditation? Only *you* know what will help because you are the expert on your pain.

THE IMMUNE SYSTEM

The presence of a reproducing virus or bacteria in your body produces an unwanted effect — you get sick. Bacteria, viruses, and parasites can cause respiratory illnesses, neurological symptoms, digestive problems, and more. The function of the immune system is to defend the body from invaders, remove damaged cells, and to remove mutant cells (such as some cancers).

A healthy immune system accomplishes this function quite well in most cases by:

- Creating barriers against viruses and bacteria that are difficult to penetrate.
- Recognizing and hunting down the bacteria or virus and killing it before it has a chance to reproduce.
- Battling to eliminate a bacteria or virus that has already started reproducing and causing symptoms.

The immune system has many jobs. It is able to produce antibodies that are specific to foreign matter that may enter the body. The antibody attaches itself to the foreign body and carries it off. The immune system retains information about that particular intruder and recognizes it if it tries to attack again at a later time.

The body is also able to recognize its own cells. When an organ transplant is performed, the body's immune system tries to destroy the new organ because it does not recognize it as its own tissue, so the patient must take immunosuppressive drugs to keep the body from rejecting the new organ. These drugs put the transplant patient at extreme risk of attack from any opportunistic virus, bacteria, or parasite that comes along.

The immune system is composed of many parts, each with its particular job:

- Skin — the body's first line of defense against invaders, it acts as a barrier.
- Nose — mucous in the nose contains a substance that combats bacteria.
- Mouth — saliva is antibacterial.
- Eyes — tears also contain a substance that combats bacteria.

If germs should make it through your defenses, they then have to contend with the major parts of the immune system which include hormones, antibodies, the lymph system, spleen, bone marrow, complement system, thymus, and white blood cells.

Lymph system: lymph is blood plasma, blood without its red cells, a clear liquid that functions to provide nutrients to the cells. Lymph also takes away the waste products of cells. When the lymph nodes are combating certain kinds of bacteria, they swell with lymph, bacteria, and the cells fighting them. After lymph filters through the lymph nodes it re-enters the blood. Swollen lymph nodes can usually be felt, and are sometimes tender.

Thymus: a glandular structure located near your heart, its main function is the production of T cells. The thymus is especially important to newborns, because if a baby's immune system is ineffective, the baby will die. An adult can live without the thymus, but will be at risk of opportunistic germs or illness.

Spleen: its main job is to filter the blood and rid it of foreign cells. It also looks for old red blood cells that need to be replaced.

Antibodies: produced by white blood cells, each antibody responds to a specific antigen (such as a bacteria, virus, or toxin). When the antibody and the antigen meet, the antibody binds to the antigen and disposes of it.

Bone marrow: produces new red and white blood cells.

Hormones: some hormones are produced by parts of the immune system. These types of hormones are called lymphokines. Some hormones in the body, the steroids and corticosteroids, actually suppress the immune system.

Complement system: a series of proteins produced in the liver, complement proteins are activated by, and work in conjunction with, antibodies. Together they cause a cell to burst and then signal phagocytes (cells that eat other cells) that a cell needs to be disposed of.

White blood cells: the most important part of the immune system, there are several different types of white blood cells that all work to seek out and destroy viruses and bacteria.

T Cells: also known as Killer T cells; have the ability to detect cells infected with a virus and destroy them.

Generally, you don't give much thought to your immune system until something causes a reaction that forces you to pay attention. For example:

- "The intact skin is the body's first line of defense." One of our nursing instructors drummed this adage into our heads years ago. When a foreign object enters the body, the immune system immediately responds to that intrusion, attacking any bacteria or virus that may have entered. When a skin wound becomes infected, the area will become inflamed and fill with pus. Inflammation and pus are proof that your immune system is working.

- The red bump that results from a bug bite is a sign that your immune system is working.

- The common cold is caused by a virus. When you get a cold, it proves that your immune system wasn't working well enough to stop the invading virus. When you get over the cold, it's proof that your immune system is back on the job. (Remember, antibiotics are not effective against a viral infection.)

- You also ingest a lot of germs when you eat. In most cases they are killed by your saliva or stomach acid. If certain germs make it through the stomach, you may develop a case of food poisoning and experience nausea, vomiting, diarrhea, and weakness. At this point you must be especially vigilant because you can quickly become dehydrated, which can debilitate you further.

Sometimes it seems the immune system has a mind of its own and can turn against you. Some examples of the immune system overreacting or working incorrectly are:

- Diabetes (type 1) — the immune system has destroyed pancreatic cells.

- Allergies — the immune system is overdoing its job, overreacting to certain substances.

- Rheumatoid arthritis — the immune system attacks the body's joints, causing pain, inflammation, swelling, and sometimes destruction of joints.

In conclusion, when your immune system is working properly, all of these systems work synergistically for optimum health. When something goes awry, the result can be fibromyalgia, CFS, multiple sclerosis, herpes, allergies, and more.

So listen to what your body is telling you. If you feel something is wrong with you, seek help and don't take no for an answer. It's up to you to get the right doctor or health care specialist to assist you with your condition.

6
CHOOSING A DOCTOR

All doctors should have at least one operation.
— Unknown

Unfortunately, many times the patient with CFS/FM will be met with a sarcastic, patronizing, insulting attitude from their doctor. We have an acronym for that type of behavior — IAIYH — It's All in Your Head. It means the doctor doesn't believe you. The doctor may think you are making up your symptoms, seeking drugs, or are just bored and want attention. So you're told that you need psychiatric help and are dismissed as though you are a wayward child. You don't need this kind of behavior from someone to whom you are paying good money. If you were treated rudely at Sears or Wal-Mart would you return? NO! You would take your business elsewhere.

You *must* find a doctor who will listen to you, believe you, and be a willing partner in your health care. The risk with this strategy is that you may get a reputation of being a "doctor shopper" and may not be taken as seriously as you should be. To counteract this view, be sure to tell the new doctor that you are looking for help, and, as yet, have been unable to find it and that you sincerely hope s/he can help you. *Never* speak ill of any other doctor you have seen to a new doctor. A valued member of our support group went to 23 different doctors and spent around $60,000 before finally, through her own research efforts, made a diagnosis on her own. She then saw a rheumatologist who gave her a proper exam, asked all the right questions, ordered all the right tests, and then came up with the correct diagnosis. They worked together as partners in her health care. This significantly reduced her stress level and she can now concentrate on her health rather than trying to convince someone that she has a legitimate health problem. *That's* the type of relationship you want and need with your own doctor.

When looking for a new doctor you should know beforehand what you want out of the relationship. What are your goals? Of course you want a doctor who is trustworthy, who believes you, respects you, is willing to work *with* you, wants to hear your opinions, encourages you to ask questions, and *wants* you to be a part of the decision-making process

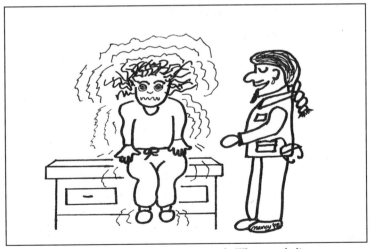

"Now accept the FACT that you are not sick. When you believe you are healthy, then you will be healthy."

regarding your health care. You also want a doctor who doesn't resent you when you ask "Why?" and you want a doctor who is willing to seek a second opinion.

Your doctor should not object when you ask, "Why are you ordering this blood work? What are you looking for? Is this test necessary? Is there anything I have to do to prepare for the test?" I also consider it important that my doctor be willing to consider my desire to explore alternative treatments and therapies such as Reiki, acupuncture, herbs, etc. Being an active participant in your health care means you have to be fairly organized and knowledgeable about your illness. This takes some time to achieve and will also require staying up-to-date on the latest information.

You must do your part in this doctor/patient relationship. You must be willing and able to share any information you have about your illness. Don't assume your doctor knows all there is to know about it. Be brief and concise. Don't bring volumes of medical books to his office and expect him to sit down and read everything you bring in. Your doctor is human and has other patients and a life. Your doctor also has a need to take care of his/her own physical and emotional needs, so please don't feel your doctor was put on this earth to minister only to you and your needs. Be reasonable about your expectations.

Ask your doctor if it's okay to bring a tape recorder when you visit and explain that this illness affects your memory. Or bring a notepad and pencil and write things down. I've found that bringing along a friend who understands this illness can be especially helpful. I have a friend who accompanies me to my doctor visits and I accompany her to hers. More than once, one of us has remembered something important the other had forgotten.

When you do go to the doctor, make sure you are well groomed. Having an unkempt or slovenly appearance may lead to a diagnosis of depression and any further possibilities will be left by the wayside.

Being organized is the key to reducing cognitive difficulties. It also aids in memory recall. This takes time but is well worth the effort. First, obtain copies of all your medical records. Make two copies so you will have a copy for yourself, one for a new doctor, and a copy in case you need to apply for Social Security Disability later on.

Review your records. If you dispute anything in your records, you have recourse. Write your "rebuttal" *on a separate sheet of paper* and include it in the record. Send a copy of your rebuttal to the doctor who wrote the disputed section and insist it be included in the original record.

Get a couple of notebooks, one to keep and one for you to bring to the new doctor. Organize the notebook into sections as you see fit. You can have a section for diagnostic tests such as blood work, x-rays, etc. Have another section for treatments tried and results obtained and one for medications tried and the results or lack of results. Make sure you include all the over-the-counter medications, herbs, supplements, etc. that you've tried. Each doctor or specialist you have seen should have a separate section. You should also have a section for your personal history and family medical history, including allergies, hereditary diseases, etc.

Be sure you list *every* symptom you have. Don't assume that by giving him the diagnosis your doctor will know all the symptoms *you* are experiencing. Also, if possible, list the dates each symptom started as well as when the medication(s) or treatment began and ended. Be as specific as possible, because if you don't write it down, you're liable to forget it and sure as shootin' you're going to be asked about it.

Now, I know this is only common sense, but it still bears repeating: each time you go to the doctor, write down the questions you want to ask beforehand. I write questions as they occur to me over time instead of waiting until just before my appointment. Doing this saves you time and will decrease the very real possibility of cognitive problems. And you won't leave the office saying, "Darn! I forgot to ask about..." This indicates to the doctor that you want to be an equal partner in managing your health.

It may seem like a lot of work, but in the long run it will be helpful to keep all of your symptoms, questions, *and* answers in a book. Getting your questions answered and keeping track of what *you* are doing will also serve to reassure you that you are once again in control of your life — *you* are in charge — not your illness. That's a very good feeling! This illness will take over your life *only if you let it!*

Now that you know what qualities you are looking for in a doctor, you have to decide what type of doctor you wish to see. Let's examine a few of the specialty practices available to you.

CHIROPRACTIC: A doctor of chiropractic medicine (DC) requires two years of undergraduate work, a four-year degree from a chiropractic college, and an internship. The theory behind chiropractic is that disease is caused by interference with nerve function due to misalignment of the spinal column, which prevents messages being transmitted to various organs and tissues. Chiropractors work by manipulating the spine to achieve wellness. Chiropractors cannot prescribe medications.

Many people in our support group have seen chiropractors and give their experience a good rating, however, for some reason they stop going and return to their primary physician. It could be that the symptoms the chiropractor can fix are lessened and they need the primary care physician to work on other symptoms. We also have many members who have *not* had a good experience with a chiropractor and even complained of symptoms worsening after treatment. The decision of whether or not to try chiropractic treatment will have to be up to you.

HOMEOPATHIC: No formal schools. Practitioners receive at least 200 hours of training and about half of all practitioners hold other medical degrees. Diseases encountered by the homeopathic practitioner are treated by drugs that, when administered in very small doses to a healthy person, will produce the symptoms of the disease being treated, which, in turn, will help you fight it.

NATUROPATHIC: A doctor of naturopathy (ND) requires a bachelor's degree and a four-year degree from a naturopathic medical school. Naturopaths treat patients without drugs or surgery by using natural methods such as light, air, water, sun, herbs, etc.

ALLOPATHIC: A doctor of medicine (MD) requires a bachelor's degree, a four-year medical degree, internship, and residency. This is the traditional western doctor who uses drugs, surgery, and other measures shown to successfully treat disease.

OSTEOPATHIC: A doctor of osteopathy, (DO) requires a bachelor's degree, a four-year osteopathic medical degree, internship, and residency. Like allopathic physicians, DOs use drugs and surgery, but osteopathic practitioners also employ manipulation of the body parts and believe that the body is continually trying to heal itself naturally and will do so if given the opportunity (good nutrition, exercise, good posture, etc.).

TRADITIONAL CHINESE MEDICINE: Many practitioners study in three-year programs. Some states allow MDs, DOs, and chiropractors to practice TCM after 200 hours of study.

REIKI: meaning "Universal Life Force" is a "hands-on" system of healing. The Reiki practitioner channels natural healing powers through touch to the person requesting it. They are not doctors and no promises of cures or pretensions of diagnosis are made. Reiki supports the feeling of well being, and, if a person feels stress or pain, the Reiki practitioner works to relieve it. Reiki is easily learned and is fast becoming accepted by traditional medical practitioners and hospitals. Other techniques, similar to Reiki, are grouped under the heading of energy therapies. Some seem to be effective. Since they don't involve drugs or invasive procedures, they are generally considered safe. Talk with your primary care doctor if you are interested in trying one of these techniques.

What I want is relief. I want to be "me" again. I want to find out what is going on with *me*, so I go to my doctor and recite my litany of woes. If I'm *lucky*, s/he believes me and we embark on a treatment plan that benefits me and makes my life more bearable.

7
LAB TESTS

As I see it, every day you do one of two things: build
health or produce disease in yourself
— Adele Davis

To make a diagnosis, rule out other possible causes of your health problems, or to monitor the effectiveness of the medications you're taking, your doctor will undoubtedly order some blood and urine tests. Here we include a list of some of what we consider to be the more common and reasonable tests that may be ordered.

COMPLETE BLOOD COUNT (CBC): The CBC is a series of tests consisting of nine different components that determine the condition of all the blood's elements. Components included in the CBC are:

- Red blood count (RBC or erythrocyte count) — The function of red blood cells is to deliver oxygen to the body's cells and remove carbon dioxide in order to prevent the build up of this waste gas. The red blood cell count is done to assess the number, the size, and shape of red blood cells. A low RBC count can indicate anemia, fluid overload, or recent hemorrhage. A high

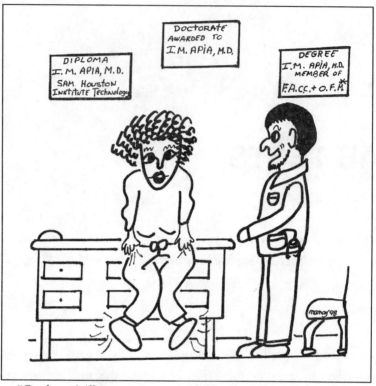

"Good news! All your tests are normal. There's nothing wrong with you.
You're in good health!"
*Fellow of American College of Clowns & Other Funny Men

RBC count may indicate primary or secondary polycythemia or dehydration. Normal RBC values differ depending on the age and sex of the patient.

- White blood count (WBC or leukocyte count) — an extremely important line of defense, the main function of white blood cells is to guard the body against infection and inflammation. A white blood count can help to determine if inflammation or infection is present, to see if further testing is needed, or to assess response to chemotherapy or radiation therapy. A high WBC can indicate infection (such as appendicitis) and with an extremely high WBC, leukemia is suspected. A low WBC indicates bone marrow depression, which may be due to viral infection, toxic reaction, or an enlarged spleen. A low white blood cell count is also seen in diseases such as influenza, typhoid fever, measles, infectious hepatitis, mononucleosis, and rubella. The normal WBC value range is 4,100-10,900/ml.

- Hemoglobin (Hgb) — about one third of each red blood cell is made up of hemoglobin. Hemoglobin contains iron and it also carries oxygen throughout the body. A hemoglobin level is obtained to determine the presence of anemia or polycythemia and to monitor response to therapy. A high hemoglobin level can be suggestive of dehydration. Persons with low hemoglobin levels will be anemic. Normal values differ depending on the age and sex of the patient.

- Hematocrit (Hct or "crit") — represents the percentage of the volume of whole blood consisting of red blood cells. Hematocrit results are used along with the hemoglobin and red blood cell count in assessing anemia as well as assessing a patient's hydration status. Red blood cells generally make up about 45 percent of the volume of whole blood, however normal values differ according to the patient's age and sex. Men generally have a higher hematocrit.

- White blood cell differential (differential or "diff") — a determination of the percentage of each of five different types of white blood cells (neutrophil, lymphocyte, monocyte, eosinophil, and basophil). Values are interpreted in relation to the overall white blood cell count. The differential helps to assess the body's response to infection, detect and identify various kinds of blood cancers, determine the stage and severity of an infection, and detect and assess the severity of an allergic reaction or parasitic infection. In manual differentials the appearance of red blood cells is also evaluated and platelet counts are estimated. Abnormal differentials are indicative of many different illnesses.

- Platelets — these sticky cells are the "glue" of the body. Their job is to stop bleeding by clumping together to "plug the leak." Some diseases cause low platelet levels, causing the patient to bleed easily and more excessively than normal. Higher platelet levels are found during pregnancy and after strenuous exercise. Higher levels are also found in bone marrow diseases and are known to contribute to heart disease and blood clotting disorders.

ARTHRITIC PANEL: Rheumatoid arthritis is an autoimmune disease, which means your immune system attacks your own body, destroying the joints. No single test can be used to diagnose rheumatoid arthritis. Diagnosis is made by evaluating your symptoms, medical history, physical examination of your joints, and lab test results.

- Erythrocyte sedimentation rate (ESR or "sed rate") — measures the rate (in millimeters) at which red blood cells fall within a calibrated tube in one hour. This is a non-specific test done to assess inflammatory response and to aid in the diagnosis of illnesses such as rheumatoid arthritis.

- Antinuclear antibodies (ANA) — this test determines the presence and amount of abnormal antibodies (autoantibodies) in the blood. While everyone has small amounts of autoantibodies, when present in higher amounts, the body's immune system overreacts by destroying its own cells because they aren't recognized as belonging in the body. This action occurs in diseases such as lupus (systemic lupus erythematosus), some viruses, and other autoimmune diseases.

- C-reactive protein (CRP) — another non-specific test that can indicate the presence of an acute infection or inflammatory process such as rheumatoid arthritis or rheumatic fever.

THYROID FUNCTION: These are the primary tests for thyroid function.

- T-3 (serum triiodothyronine) — aids in the diagnosis of hypo and hyperthyroidism, and to monitor response to treatment of hypothyroidism. T-3 levels closely rise and fall in tandem with T-4 levels and it takes an expert to interpret the results when one rises and the other doesn't. Don't attempt to figure this out on your own; leave it to your doctor.

- T-4 (serum thyroxine) — aids in diagnosing hypo and hyperthyroidism, monitor response to treatment with antithyroid medication in hyperthyroidism, and to monitor response to replacement therapy in hypothyroidism.

- TSH (thyroid stimulating hormone) — this test is performed to distinguish between primary and secondary hypothyroidism and to monitor effectiveness of treatment. Again, the results should be left to the experts to interpret, as there are many variables to be taken into account.

BASIC METABOLIC PANEL: The basic metabolic panel consists of a combination of elements used to evaluate body metabolism. A typical metabolic panel measures the levels of sodium, potassium, calcium, chloride, carbon dioxide, glucose, blood urea nitrogen (BUN), and creatinine in the blood — all of which are responsible for helping maintain a healthy body.

- Sodium — an electrolyte that is responsible for fluid balance in the body, it is also responsible for neuromuscular, kidney, and adrenal functioning. Low values can result from excessive diarrhea, vomiting, and sweating.

- Potassium — an electrolyte essential to homeostasis, potassium is responsible for regulating electrical conduction in the muscles and in maintaining acid/base (pH) balance. Potassium correlates with sodium in that if there is an increase in one, there is a decrease in the other. Potassium depletion can occur rapidly because the body has no way to store it. High levels of potassium can occur in cases of severe burns or myocardial infarct.

- Calcium — approximately 98 percent of the body's store of calcium is found in the bones and teeth. Calcium is responsible for skeletal growth and stability and for the regulation of neuromuscular action. When blood levels of calcium fall, calcium from the teeth and bones will be leeched to restore normal levels in the blood.

- Chloride — an electrolyte important for maintaining the acid/base balance in the body. Low levels lead to slow respirations and hypertonicity of the muscles. High levels lead to fast respirations, weakness, and stupor, all of which can possibly lead to coma.

- Carbon dioxide (CO_2) — Your body oxidizes carbon atoms in food to make CO_2, which is then excreted by the lungs. CO_2 levels are good indicators of the body's acidity or alkalinity. With conditions such as pneumonia or emphysema, abnormal, slow, shallow respirations lead to a rise in carbon dioxide levels and metabolic alkalosis occurs. Conditions such as diabetic acidosis, kidney failure, or hyperventilation cause CO_2 levels to fall, creating a state of metabolic acidosis.

- Glucose — the main source of energy for the body's cells, glucose is formed through conversion of the carbohydrates you eat. High glucose levels are found in diabetes, pancreatitis, and patients with poor diets. Low levels are found in cases of increased insulin production by the pancreas and hypothyroidism.

- Blood urea nitrogen (BUN) — a waste product of protein metabolism by the liver and excreted by the kidneys, BUN is an indicator of kidney function and also aids in assessing the quality of hydration.

- Creatinine — another component to assess kidney function, creatinine is a waste product of muscle metabolism.

ROUTINE URINALYSIS (UA): Used to screen for urinary tract disorders and assess kidney function, the urine is evaluated for color, odor, and whether the sample is clear or cloudy. A chemical test strip is used to quantify specific gravity, glucose, and pH (acidity or alkalinity). A microscopic exam is performed to check for the presence of red or white blood cells, yeast, parasites, or crystals.

IRON STUDIES: Used to check the oxygen carrying capacity of the blood.

- Serum iron, total iron binding capacity (tibc), and ferritin: — these tests give a pretty good indication of the amount of iron in your blood and are an important aid in the diagnosis of high or low iron states. Low iron levels lead to conditions such as anemia.

VIRAL TESTING: Viruses are submicroscopic organisms that cause infections and are able to replicate *only* in living cells. Viruses do their dirty work by destroying, maiming, and killing most of the cells they infect, damaging the immune system, lowering your resistance to disease and infection, and are the cause of many different illnesses. Viruses change the DNA of the cells they infect and can cause inflammation that damages organs. These are mean, nasty little fellas! Viruses are responsible for diseases such as AIDS, cold sores, chicken pox, measles, influenza, and some types of cancer.

Viral testing can detect the presence or absence of those viral conditions as well as Epstein-Barr virus, cytomegalovirus (CMV), hepatitis, human papillomavirus (HPV or genital warts), and influenza.

Viral testing may soon also be available to screen for CFS as well. A zoonotic virus has been identified as possibly being responsible for CFS. This virus was originally found to occur in swine, and later in other animals and finally in humans.

The National CFIDS Foundation explained it this way in a press release dated May 31, 2006:

Potential Animal (Zoonotic) Virus Identified in Patients with Chronic Fatigue Syndrome, Multiple Sclerosis, and Epilepsy

Recent independent scientific research funded by the National CFIDS Foundation, Inc. (NCF) of Needham, MA provided preliminary confirmation of a new virus identified in patients with Chronic Fatigue Syndrome. The Foundation's medical research dovetails with that completed to date by Cryptic Afflictions, LLC, a private company.

Dr. Steven K. Robbins, virologist and chief executive officer of Cryptic Afflictions, LLC has discovered a major neuropathogen identified as an RNA virus designated as Cryptovirus. Substantial clinical and molecular evidence indicates that this virus is involved in the development of neurological disorders that include Chronic Fatigue Syndrome (CFS), also known as Myalgic Encephalomyelitis (ME) by the World Health Organization, Multiple Sclerosis (MS), and Idiopathic Epilepsy of unknown cause.

According to the company, "This previously undetected virus appears to be of significant importance to researchers looking for a cure to Multiple Sclerosis and many other neurological illnesses. Antibodies to the newly discovered virus were found in the cerebrospinal fluid and blood of over 90 percent of the patients tested with Multiple Sclerosis. It is believed that this newly discovered virus may prove to be responsible for a host of neurological disorders. Tests are currently being prepared for tissue samples of lesions within the brains of patients with Multiple Sclerosis. This will be the final round of tests before approaching the FDA for approval of the diagnostic tests."

Dr. Robbins' evidence includes the presence of virus-specific antibodies in the serum and cerebrospinal fluid of patients suffering from these disorders, the ability of the virus to cause virtually identical disease in experimentally infected animals, and nucleotide sequence data that indicates that the virus is pandemic and represents a single virus species much like measles.

A recently published medical journal article suggests that Cryptovirus is most similar to Parainfluenza Virus-5, a rubulavirus in the paramyxovirus family. Another rubulavirus related to Cryptovirus and Parainfluenza Virus-5, that has gained national attention for its large outbreak, is the mumps virus. Rubulavirus infections have been associated with encephalitis, meningitis, orchitis, inflammation of the testicles or ovaries, spontaneous abortion and deafness.

The NCF has conducted its own preliminary research into the potential role of Cryptovirus and Parainfluenza Virus-5 in Chronic Fatigue Syndrome. Professor Alan Cocchetto, Medical Director for the Foundation stated, "Our own funded research first confirmed the lack of a vital protein, known as Stat-1 in the blood of patients with Chronic Fatigue Syndrome. Stat-1 plays an indispensable role in immunity. Without this protein, patients are unable to effectively fight viral and bacterial infections. Thus, the next logical question to be answered was 'Could a virus be causing this Stat-1 depletion?'" Cocchetto continued, "Parainfluenza Virus-5 is a virus that had to be seriously considered as a possible piece of this medical puzzle because it directly targets and destroys the Stat-1 protein. Gail Kansky, President of the NCF stated, "Once we determined the status of Stat-1 in patient blood samples, we knew that we had to look for possible evidence of Parainfluenza Virus-5 infection. It was during this phase of our own research that we actually learned of Dr. Steven Robbins' discovery of Cryptovirus specific antibody reactivity in patients with CFS." Dr. Robbins has tested fifty-six serum specimens from patients who had been diagnosed with CFS along with eleven matching cerebrospinal fluid samples obtained from physicians in Brisbane and Southeast Queensland. Dr. Robbins had determined that ninety-six percent of the blood samples and ninety-one percent of the spinal fluid samples tested positively for Cryptovirus specific antibodies in these CFS patients.

The National CFIDS Foundations' own research began to dovetail with that of Dr. Robbins. Scientists funded by the Foundation performed numerous tests for Parainfluenza Virus-5 that included antibody as well as PCR specific probes. Antibody testing provided some initial hints, however a PCR specific probe picked up the infection in a former patient of David S. Bell, M.D. and Paul R. Cheney, Ph.D., M.D., both considered well known specialists in the field of Chronic Fatigue Syndrome. Kansky commented, "Though our funded research continues in diagnostic testing, our findings have served to highlight the important work of Dr. Robbins and the role of Cryptovirus and Parainfluenza Virus-5 infection in CFS."

— Reprinted with permission
National CFIDS Foundation, Gail Kansky, President.

We continue to hope that ongoing research will help provide a diagnostic test for CFS and other related diseases.

8
TRADITIONAL THERAPIES

Make your own recovery the first priority in your life.
— Robin Norvin

After all the months, maybe years, of suffering and thinking you're crazy or a "wimp," your doctor has finally made the correct diagnosis for you. It may seem strange, but you are relieved! At last a name has been put to your miseries. You have been validated. Your doctor believes you and believes that there *is* an illness called CFS or fibromyalgia! You can feel the load on your shoulders lighten and you feel less stress. But you also still feel lousy. So, what can you expect from "traditional" medicine?

Your doctor will most likely start you off with a combination of medications in order for you to get some good, restorative sleep — essential for pain relief! He or she may have you start on a gentle stretching and reconditioning program. A sensible suggestion — *if* you have fibromyalgia, that is. Fibromyalgia patients usually respond well to exercise, whereas exercise can put the CFS patient over the edge and make symptoms worse. You will be told to follow a sensible diet; that's a given for any illness. You may even be told to get some physical therapy or aquatic therapy. Most likely your doctor will write you a prescription for a very low dose of an antidepressant, often Elavil (amitriptyline) and possibly a muscle relaxant such as Flexeril (cyclobenzaprine). These are good suggestions and they often work very well in the beginning. It's always best to start with the basics.

Being the curious person you are you'll want to know why particular therapies are suggested by your doctor. Especially, why take an antidepressant? You're not depressed. Did your doctor maybe go a little too far ordering an antidepressant? No! And here's why — antidepressants help alleviate pain by their action on serotonin and norepinephrine in the pain pathways in the brain. Antidepressants usually take from four to six weeks to begin to take effect. Antidepressants are not addicting but your dosage may need to be adjusted periodically, as your body's need for the medication may vary.

The use of muscle relaxants is obvious. When you're under stress, such as that caused by being in pain, your muscles tense up, causing more pain. When the muscles relax, the pain goes away. Used together, the two drugs work synergistically, allowing you to get the quality sleep required to rebuild your body's energy store, making it possible for you to do all the good things you should be doing for yourself. Underconditioned muscles are also stressed muscles. That's why your doctor is likely to recommend stretching and gentle exercise, possibly including physical or aquatic therapy as part of a reconditioning program.

Physical therapy can also help restore loss of function that you may have experienced due to the symptoms of your illness. Physical therapy is very gentle and relaxing and helps to decrease stress while it gradually builds strength and endurance, one baby step at a time. Perhaps one of the most important functions of the physical therapist is patient education. The motto of the physical therapist (at least the ones I've had contact with) is "If it hurts to do it, then don't do it." Treatment usually consists of massage, joint manipulation, and teaching the use of mechanical aids, among other modalities. One modality sometimes offered is aquatic therapy, a series of exercises done in a heated pool. The warmth and buoyancy of the water allow patients to perform exercises easier than they could on land by decreasing the stress placed on the body, allowing for easier movement. The warm water feels good, relaxing those tense muscles and increasing blood flow to the affected areas.

If you have pain, analgesic medication will be prescribed for you.

It is important that you develop a trusting partnership with your doctor by honestly reporting your progress, or lack of it, and always taking your prescription medication as prescribed. If you feel you need more or less of a medication, talk with your prescribing doctor rather than changing what you are taking on your own.

These are great treatment plans, and the chances of them bringing you relief are excellent. However, nothing lasts forever, so be prepared to continue to use what you learn and to make a few changes now and then since the course of action that is best for you may change with time.

9
ALTERNATIVE THERAPIES

We don't believe in rheumatism or true love until after
the first attack
— Marie von Eschenbach

There are many alternative therapies that may be effective for you. Some that you can do on your own, such as meditation, are almost certainly safe. Others may be better undertaken only after you discus them with your doctor. In any case, if you have a good doctor, he or she should be happy to discus the possible therapies to find the ones that will work best for you.

Meditation —a relaxing, wonderful way to reduce stress that leaves one feeling calm and peaceful. Lisa has had success with this treatment and is very pleased with the results. On the other hand, I find meditation to be stressful because my brain won't shut down. My thoughts race and I start thinking about everything but meditating. Everyone responds differently, however, so it's definitely worth a try. Anything you can do to reduce stress is good for you.

Diversion therapy — involves thinking about and concentrating on something other than your pain. In other words, try to forget about the pain by wholeheartedly immersing yourself in some other endeavor. This treatment is effective only when the pain is not severe. Redirecting and refocusing your concerns and energies by getting involved with something that interests you, such as a hobby, a really good book, a puzzle — all of these can temporarily help take your mind off your pain.

Relaxation — it sounds easy, but conscious relaxation really takes a lot of practice and concentration. Wear comfortable clothing, lie down, stretch, and breathe deeply a few times. Be aware of your breathing throughout this therapy. Your breathing should be calm and easy with an occasional deep cleansing breath.

To begin the relaxation exercise, concentrate first on totally relaxing your feet. When this is accomplished, move on to relaxing your ankles, then the calves of your legs, the knees, the thighs, etc. Concentrate on your breathing and on relaxing each body part. Don't move on until each part (and the parts before) are totally relaxed.

Quite often you'll find you've tensed up again. If a part becomes tense again, go back to that point and start over. With practice you can do it, and when you do accomplish total relaxation you will feel so-o-o good! The key is to do the exercise when you know you won't be interrupted and when there are no other demands being made of you. I usually do this at bedtime. Many people find that this therapy works beautifully to reduce stress and tension as well as promoting relaxation and sleep.

Biofeedback — with biofeedback you learn how to gain conscious control of regulating body processes such as breathing, blood pressure, temperature, and heart rate. The patient is first taught a relaxation exercise and how to identify circumstances that trigger symptoms.

When using biofeedback, you must commit to practice every day and accept responsibility for maintaining your own health. This treatment works. I don't know exactly why or how, but I have watched in rapt fascination as one of my group members used it on herself. She had been shaky and unbalanced and was getting worse with each step she took. Then she stopped, closed her eyes, and concentrated as our whole group watched. After a few minutes she opened her eyes, smiled at us, and walked away without help as if nothing had happened.

Reflexology — involves applying pressure to certain points on the hands and feet, specifically the "tender points" that are thought to be linked to specific organs in the body. Reflexology is used in an effort to decrease stress to that particular part of the body.

It's important to remember that this treatment is to be used *in addition* to medical treatment and not as the only treatment. At the end of a treatment session you should feel relaxed and free of stress. The indicator of the success of the treatment is how long that relaxed feeling lasts. In my humble opinion, reflexology probably helps for a while and may well help reduce stress. However there are many ways to reduce stress without spending money to do it. I would equate this treatment with massage.

Cranial-sacral therapy — involves gentle massage of the skull and spine in order to move the liquid that surrounds them. This treatment affects the whole body and generates a feeling of general well being and a significant reduction in stress. Not surprisingly, this therapy relieves headaches and jaw and neck pain, which are areas most affected by stress.

It's quite possible your insurance company will cover this therapy with an order from your doctor, but do some research and check with them first. This is another treatment Lisa highly recommends because it has given her measurable pain and stress relief.

Acupressure/acupuncture — these two treatments are very similar. In acupressure, pressure is applied to certain acupuncture points on the body. In acupuncture, very fine, sterile needles are inserted at certain points on the body.

Feelings about these therapies are mixed. Some people that have tried one or the other of these treatments did not experience either improvement or decline of symptoms. Lisa has had great success, though. Unfortunately, these treatments may be too expensive because many insurance companies do not cover them.

Cognitive behavior therapy (CBT) — although symptoms of chronic fatigue syndrome or fibromyalgia are physical, CBT can help a person cope with the symptoms of our physical illness. Our symptoms are *physical* — we can't "think" them away, but we can use our thought processes to find more effective ways to cope with the pain we have. No one wants to be ill. It's not fun and it costs a lot of money.

Transcutaneous electrical nerve stimulator (TENS) — is a machine that is attached to the body in order to transmit electrical impulses that interrupt and redirect pain signals from the brain. I have used a TENS unit and find the results to be fast and very effective, but unfortunately, the results are fleeting.

Magnet therapy — some believe that magnets have a beneficial effect when placed on certain parts of the body (wrist, feet, back) for such varied problems as back pain or carpal tunnel syndrome. People who deal in facts and science are extremely critical of the claims made by magnet therapy proponents. Because there is no scientific evidence of efficacy and the use of magnets is so widespread, FDA regulations prohibit the promotion of magnets as an effective treatment for any condition.

If you decide to try this therapy and you have a cardiac pacemaker or an Interstim device in your buttock *check with your doctor first*, as the magnet may interfere with their functioning.

Reiki — means "universal life force" and is a hands-on treatment to release energy within the body, allowing the energy to flow into the areas that need it. Reiki is not used to treat illness, but as an adjunct to medical treatment. It can help decrease nausea caused by chemotherapy and helps to reduce stress and anxiety.

I heartily believe in Reiki and practice on myself. You may be practicing it on yourself without knowing it. By this I mean that when you hurt somewhere (headache, stomachache, bump on the leg or arm, a bleeding cut, or minor burn) what do you do? You instinctively put your hand(s) on the painful area and hold that area for a while. As the area is healing, you may feel a slight tingle in your fingers and soon the area feels better. That's Reiki.

If you have an opportunity to take a Reiki course or to have a Reiki treatment, do it! It's a wonderful healing art and can even be performed with success on animals. Many hospitals offer this before and after surgery and have great results with patients' recovery.

Massage therapy — consists of rubbing and kneading the body in a systematic and therapeutic manner that is very relaxing for many people. I have a problem with massage because it hurts me to be touched, making this a stressful treatment for me. However, many people, including Lisa, swear that massage can be very healing. Lisa makes it a point to treat herself monthly to a full-body massage and finds it quite soothing.

Imagery — is accomplished by imagining yourself in a special, pleasant place or picturing yourself as being "well." Imagery is also used to "combat" illness. I have heard of people imagining their cancer (or other cause of illness) as a hated object and themselves as a ferocious tiger or bear. They then imagine that they are devouring or beating that hated object. They continue with this imagery until the hated object is eliminated. This is done as often as it's felt to be necessary. This type of therapy can help give you a feeling of power over your illness. Hey, whatever works!

Self-hypnosis — a method of inducing in yourself a state of calm, relaxed passivity where you become responsive to suggestion (if you so choose). It's important to understand that a person who has been hypnotized *will not* do something in a hypnotized state that they would not do in a wakeful, non-hypnotized state.

Physical therapy — can involve massage, moist heat, ice, ultrasound, and specific exercises to increase strength or flexibility, among other modalities.

Myofascial release — is not for the faint of heart. It hurts. It involves a deep massage where the muscles and the tissues surrounding them are grabbed, lifted, and maneuvered around.

Trigger point injection — saline solution, lidocaine, and sometimes steroids are injected into the painful areas by a doctor and then those areas are massaged.

Hydrotherapy — involves soaking in a hot tub, Jacuzzi, warm bath, or warm pool. Water therapy seems to be one of the best forms of therapy.

Occupational therapy — not strictly for work related problems, OT also helps patients with activities of daily living.

Pet therapy — having a pet can lower your blood pressure, improve your state of mind, and give you a feeling of self-worth. An animal does not judge you, and sitting quietly while petting your cat or dog can significantly lower your stress level. Also, having a pet to care for gets you up and moving in order to fulfill their needs for exercise and feeding.

Herb therapy — many drugs come from herbs or plants of one sort or another. If you doubt the potency or effectiveness of plants, remember that foxglove is used in making digitalis (a heart regulating drug) and that marijuana is also an herb. Everyone knows that marijuana works. Please check with your doctor before you use any kind of herb. Many have significant interaction with other medication your may be taking,

Aromatherapy — consists of using aromatic essential oils from plants added to products to be inhaled or applied to the skin to produce different effects.

Ayurveda — in this holistic form of medicine from India, it is believed that illness stems from the way you live your life and how you react to what life throws at you.

Healing arts — basically, if it makes you feel good then it must be good for you. For example, do you like music? Dancing? Creating? Writing? Do you like comedy? How do you feel when you watch a ballet, write a poem, or have a good laugh? You feel good, don't you? At least for a while. *That's* healing arts.

Chiropractic — treatment consists of manipulating the spine to bring it into correct alignment. Sometimes heat and ultrasound are also used. Chiropractic treatment is considered safe when performed by an experienced practitioner.

Some of my support group members have used chiropractors for years and have been happy with the results. Others have tried it and swear that they were worse after treatment. You must do your homework before seeing a chiropractor, just as you would any health professional. Get a referral from someone you trust. Make an appointment to meet and talk to the doctor before treatment. Then it's a personal call as to whether you'd like to try it.

Homeopathic medicine — based on the theory of "a hair of the dog that bit you," practitioners believe that if a substance will cause a symptom in a healthy person then a very small amount of that substance will cure the same symptom in a sick person. This is similar to immuno-therapy treatment for allergies that involves injecting tiny, gradually increased doses of an allergen over a period of time in order to build tolerance.

Homeopathic remedies are used for treating minor injuries, cuts, and scrapes. Homeopathic treatments are *not* deemed appropriate for serious illnesses. Some critics of homeopathy claim that any relief gained from using homeopathic remedies is the result of a placebo effect. However, some people I have great admiration and respect for have seen homeo-pathic doctors and are more than pleased with the results. Again, do your research, find a reputable practitioner, ask a lot of questions, and talk to others who have been happy with their homeopathic doctor. Then decide.

Naturopathic medicine — Naturopaths share similar educational training as allopathic doctors and use the same diagnostic techniques such as x-rays and lab tests, but naturopathy is a prevention-based style of medicine which uses botanicals, nutrition, and lifestyle counseling to manage health and treat illness.

Osteopathic medicine — doctors of osteopathy (DOs) have the same type of medical training and function the same as the medical doctor (MD), but DOs also use natural remedies and manual therapy in an effort to help the body heal itself. If you are interested in pursuing alternative therapies, it might make sense to have a DO as your primary care physician instead of an MD.

Traditional Chinese medicine — is based on the belief that to maintain good health, your yin and yang must be in balance. If they're not, it means there is a disturbance in your life and your body experiences some sort of dysfunction or disease. People who practice traditional Chinese medicine use many herbal remedies in their treatments.

I was once told that the Chinese have a unique relationship with their doctors — they pay them when they're well and stop paying them when they become sick. Hmm-m-m-m. That means Chinese doctors have a better financial reward when they have healthy patients while Western doctors earn more (much, much more) when their patients are sick. Something to think about…

Try whatever practitioner or modality sounds good to you. It may help — it may not. It may help for only a short while or it may be just what you need. Whatever you decide, be sure to talk it over with your primary care physician first. If you have the right physician, the two of you will be able to work together to find the best treatment plan for whatever happens.

10
MEDICATIONS

*It is my opinion that we are here to amuse the patient
while his body heals itself.*
— *Unknown*

There are many medications prescribed for and taken by the person with CFS with the ultimate goal of promoting good, restorative sleep patterns and eliminating or controlling pain.

You will hear a lot about the need for good, restorative sleep and there's good reason for it. While you are sleeping, you're not expending much energy and your body is restoring itself, promoting healing. Many classes of drugs are used to reach these goals of promoting good sleep and pain control. Some examples include medications for Parkinson's disease, anti-seizure medications, antianxiety drugs, antidepressants, NSAIDS, opioids, and more. It may take some time to hit upon the right medication or combination of medications that works best for you. You must give any new medication you try a good and fair trial. Some medications can take two to four weeks or more before any improvement in your symptoms occurs. You should also understand that a drug that works well for one person may not work for another.

Again, please remember to keep a *written* record of each medication you try and what your results are. We know that remembering things is a problem for most of us. Just don't forget where you put the information!

You should make the Girl Scout motto, "Be Prepared" yours as well. You can be prepared by having a well-stocked medicine cabinet.

The following items represent examples of what the person with CFS should keep on hand for themselves *and* their healthy family.

OVER THE COUNTER (OTC) MEDICATIONS

- Aspirin or Tylenol (acetaminophen) for pain or fever. Do *not* give aspirin to children under the age of 18 years because of the danger of Reye's syndrome, a serious, potentially deadly condition that damages the liver and brain.

- An antihistamine, decongestant, and expectorant for symptoms of cold, allergies, or cough.

- Aspirin, ibuprofen, or other non-steroidal anti-inflammatory drugs (NSAID) for pain, swelling, or inflammation.

- Antacids for upset stomach, heartburn, or acid indigestion.

MEDICAL SUPPLIES

- Syrup of ipecac for accidental poisoning. (Always check with Poison Control before administering syrup of ipecac — it is not appropriate for all poisonings.)

- A mild antibacterial soap or dilution of household hydrogen peroxide for cleansing wounds.

- Antibacterial ointment (like Neosporin) for minor cuts and scrapes. Do NOT use Neosporin if you have a latex allergy.
- Sunscreen with SPF 15 or higher to prevent sunburn.
- Aloe or topical anesthetic (cream or ointment ending with "caine"), or that old standby Noxzema, work well for relief of sunburn.
- Calamine lotion or hydrocortisone cream for use after exposure to poison ivy or other skin irritants. Soaking in a lukewarm bath with either baking soda or colloidal oatmeal added can also soothe irritated skin.
- Hand cream to soothe dry skin
- Thermometer
- A special, calibrated spoon, cup, or dropper to use for measuring liquid medicines. *Do not* use a kitchen spoon; it is not an accurate measure.
- Band-Aids of different sizes and shapes, sterile gauze pads, roll bandages, and adhesive tape for wound care.
- Scissors
- Tweezers to remove splinters and other foreign bodies from the skin. (Hint: A piece of duct tape placed against the splinter and then pulled away may be all you need to remove a superficial splinter. Try this before tweezers if the splinter is not deeply embedded.)
- Ace bandages of various sizes
- Rubbing alcohol (70% isopropyl alcohol)
- Antibacterial hand wipes
- Ice bag
- Humidifier

- Heating pad
- Cotton swabs

Your pharmacist is your best friend when it comes to medications, both prescription and over the counter. Make sure you tell your pharmacist about any and all medications you are taking, including herbs, vitamins or other supplements, etc. We strongly urge you to act responsibly and sensibly when medication is involved. *ALWAYS* use the same pharmacy. This advice may save your life. By using only one pharmacy, you can be assured that your medication record and history is complete and accurate. When a new drug is ordered, your pharmacist will know if there are any contraindications based on any known allergies or interactions with other meds you are currently taking.

Being a member of your health team means that you must be willing to put forth the effort to understand, appreciate, and become knowledge-able about your medications. You should know the name, prescribed dosage, frequency, and duration for each medication, as well as when

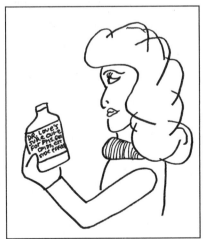

"Side effects: nausea; irritable bowel; irritable bladder; muscle pain or twitching; sleep disturbance; headache, fatigue; memory/cognitive impairment; numbness & tingling; dry skin/eyes..." How will I know if it works?

and how you should take it. You should understand what to expect from each medication, including its intended effect, possible side effects, if there is anything to avoid while taking the drug, whether there is a generic version, and if a generic form would be all right for you to take.

Be sure you know how to store your medications and what you should do if you forget to take a dose. Always let your prescribing doctor and pharmacist know if you are pregnant or trying to become pregnant, or if you are breastfeeding. Understand whether you should avoid driving or operating dangerous machinery while taking your medication. Act responsibly.

Along with medications, lifestyle changes should be part of your treatment regimen. Eat healthy foods, stop smoking, and reduce stress. In other words, be nice to yourself. Know your body and its usual state and reactions so that if a new or different symptom or reaction occurs, you will be aware of it and be able to discuss it with your doctor. Know what side effects are possible with each new medication you are prescribed. Should you experience a new symptom, let your doctor know.

A good health care consumer does not insist on a pill to cure every problem. For example, you see your doctor for symptoms of a cold. Having a cold is no fun, so you ask for an antibiotic. Now, you learned earlier that a cold is a virus and that viruses do not respond to antibiotics, so you're wasting your money and risking unwanted side effects by taking something will not make your cold go away. Due to overuse and sometimes-inappropriate use, antibiotics are fast becoming ineffective, as the "bugs" are getting stronger and more resistant to the current generation of antibiotics. Antibiotic use also carries a risk of causing problems such as yeast infections. And that condition is no fun at all!

Next time you get a cold try following the sensible route:

- Don't pressure your doctor for an antibiotic

- Get lots of rest
- Drink plenty of fluids
- Eat healthy foods
- Use a vaporizer
- Use Kleenex rather than cloth handkerchiefs
- Rub some Mentholatum on your chest, and maybe a little under your nose to relieve congestion

When taking a new drug be responsible and use common sense. Read the label each time you take the drug. Don't take any medication in the dark. Turn the light on so you can see, and put on your glasses if needed. Store your medications properly. Most should be stored in a cool, dry place (not in the medicine cabinet in a hot, steamy bathroom). Do not put meds in a bottle that was previously used for something else or mix several different drugs together in the same bottle. Properly dispose of any medications that are out of date. (Every bottle is labeled with an expiration date.) Use all medications *as directed.* If the dose seems to be too much or not enough, talk to your doctor before adjusting the dose yourself.

When your doctor prescribes a *new* medication, ask if samples are available. Ask if it's okay to start with a smaller dose and then work your way up if necessary. When filling a new prescription, tell the pharmacist you want only enough for a few days so you can see if the drug agrees with you. By doing this you won't waste a lot of money on a medication that doesn't work, or, worse yet, causes an allergic or other adverse reaction. If the drug works as it should, then you can have the rest of the prescription filled.

The medications used to treat chronic fatigue syndrome are many and varied. They range from over the counter (OTC) medications for pain like Advil to heavy-duty narcotics such as morphine. The choice of which medications to use depends on many factors: severity of pain, frequency of pain, pain location, other medications being taken, reactions to medications, what other medications have been tried, and the age, weight, and medical history of the patient. Remember, what works for one person may not work for another.

Unfortunately, the medications that work the best for moderate to severe pain, the opiates, are rarely prescribed, and when they are, they are not prescribed in an adequate dose. The reason for this is that doctors — and patients — are afraid of addiction. The patient does not want to become addicted and the doctor doesn't want to lose his license.

Psychological addiction to opiates occurs rarely when they are used properly to treat pain. Psychological addiction results when the drug is used *compulsively and uncontrollably*, often for the euphoria ("rush") that opiates can cause, and harm to the user results. This is not to say that using opiates properly is without problems. Opiates can cause physical dependence and, if the drug is stopped suddenly, symptoms of withdrawal (which generally last just a few days and are similar to symptoms of the flu) will then occur. Withdrawal from an opiate is not medically dangerous for most people and hospitalization is not usually necessary. If tapered off slowly — under the direction of the prescribing doctor who knows the person's specific health situation — there will usually be no signs or symptoms of withdrawal.

We include here some of the many groups or classifications of medications used to treat the symptoms of chronic fatigue syndrome and fibromyalgia. Specific dosages are not included, as dosage will vary with each patient and their particular medical condition.

ANALGESICS

Tylenol (acetaminophen; known as paracetamol outside the USA) does a terrific job of relieving pain. Caffeine enhances its effects. It is *not* an anti-inflammatory so it will not be effective for the pain of most arthritis, although it often works well for pain in osteoarthritis. Discuss dosage with your doctor, as overdose is possible and can lead to liver damage. You can't live without a liver, and symptoms of overdose are not seen until late in the process. Alcohol increases the danger, so DO NOT USE ALCOHOL WHILE TAKING THIS DRUG. Discuss this with your physician and your pharmacist.

Imitrex (sumatriptan) is one of many "triptans" and is prescribed for treating severe, crippling migraine headaches. Most patients get relief from taking it.

Non-steroidal anti-inflammatory drugs (NSAIDs) (sometimes referred to simply as anti-inflammatories) are often used for pain caused by inflammation, as in arthritis. While NSAIDs are anti-inflammatory, they are also analgesic and antipyretic, so they can work on your arthritis, lessen mild to moderate pain, and relieve a fever. Full therapeutic effect may take two to four weeks.

Because the main complaint with any NSAID is stomach upset, this medication should be taken with food. If taken long term, be aware of the possibility of gastrointestinal bleeding, and be aware that dark, tarry stools or "coffee ground" vomitus are signs of a gastrointestinal bleed.

Some NSAIDs, called COX-2 inhibitors, work by blocking the enzyme pathway so that stomach upset and damage is prevented. *Do not combine NSAIDs (including aspirin or other salicylates)* because the negative side effects add up with each of the drugs.

NSAIDs include trademark drugs such as Advil and Motrin (ibuprofen), Indocin (indomethacin), Naprosyn (naproxen), Relafen (nabumetone), and Feldene (piroxicam).

NARCOTICS

By far the most beneficial drugs used for severe pain *when used and prescribed appropriately*, narcotics work by binding with opiate receptors in the brain to change the perception and emotional response to pain. Narcotics should be taken before the pain becomes too severe and should be taken with food. Narcotics are very helpful for the relief of severe pain, but they carry some very serious responsibilities and possible unwanted side effects, primarily that they can become addictive.

Be sure your doctor knows your complete history and what other medications you are taking (and have taken). Let him know of any changes in your physical or psychological condition. Possible side effects of narcotics include sedation, dizziness, risk of seizures, nausea, vomiting, etc. Two significant and common side effects of the ongoing use (beyond a few weeks) of opiates are constipation and depression.

Physical addiction to opiates is a risk whenever they are used for whatever reason, including the treatment of pain, for more than several weeks. However, if an opiate is the most appropriate treatment for the pain, addiction issues become secondary. *Without exception,* opiates should be taken exactly as prescribed. If pain is not adequately relived, it may be tempting to take more than prescribed, but *never* do so for two good reasons: first, the "extra" pain may be a sign of a new, different — and possibly life-threatening — problem requiring evaluation and appropriate treatment rather than being "masked" by extra pain medication, and, second, communication with your prescribing doctor enhances the quality of the medical care you receive — and the mutual trust necessary for you and your doctor to work together on your problems. Talk with your doctor rather than taking more pain medication (opiates or other analgesic) than has been prescribed.

Some of the narcotics used to treat chronic fatigue syndrome and fibromyalgia include Vicodin (hydrocodone), Darvocet (Darvon and acetaminophen), OxyContin (oxycodone hydrochloride), Percocet (oxycodone with acetaminophen), and Ultracet (tramadol with acetaminophen)

Pain patches contain lidoderm and other narcotics are becoming popular in place of pills or injection. Duragesic (a fentanyl transdermal patch), is one example. By placing the patch on the skin directly over the pain site, gastrointestinal side effects are avoided. Some patients may experience irritation at the site of the patch.

Transdermal narcotics are *very* strong medications. The person using a patch MUST learn all they can about the drug and its possible side effects, and they MUST be observant and know their body well to be able to identify any unwanted changes that may take place.

Because opiates are powerful medications with abuse potential and with possible serious effects if taken in overdose, your supply must be kept in a secure place, safe from robbers and from unintentional use by children and other vulnerable persons.

TRICYCLIC ANTIDEPRESSANTS

This group of medications works by increasing levels of serotonin in the brain. Low serotonin levels are common in the person with chronic fatigue syndrome and fibromyalgia. Tricyclic antidepressants (TCAs) help control pain and promote sleep, and when prescribed for the purpose of relieving pain, they are prescribed in smaller doses than when prescribed for primary depression. TCAs should be taken at night for their sedative qualities. Possible side effects include dry mouth, drowsiness, morning hangover, weight gain, and, occasionally, anxiety. Some common TCAs prescribed for chronic fatigue syndrome and fibromyalgia are Elavil (amitriptyline), Pamelor (nortriptyline), and Norpramin (desipramine).

Although not a tricyclic, trazodone is an antidepressant that has similar actions, benefits, and possible side effects, and is often used to promote sleep.

Tricyclic antidepressants and trazodone may take up to four to eight weeks to significantly relieve pain, once an effective dose has been reached. However, their effect to promote sleep may occur much sooner, sometimes after the first dose.

SELECTIVE SEROTONIN RE-UPTAKE INHIBITORS (SSRIs)

SSRIs are antidepressants that boost serotonin levels and help to keep serotonin available longer. SSRIs are used to help manage fatigue, cognitive impairment, and secondary depression associated with fibromyalgia. Take an SSRI in the morning at the same time every day. It can take up to four to six weeks for the full effect of the medication to be recognized.

AVOID alcohol when taking these medications as they increase alcohol's central nervous system effects. AVOID smoking because it decreases the medication effects. AVOID St. John's wort, an OTC herbal with antidepressant qualities because it contains variable amounts of SSRI-like compounds which, when combined with a prescription SSRI antidepressant, frequently cause adverse effects.. However, tricyclic antidepressants such as Elavil can work synergistically with an SSRI to provide greater relief. Some of the possible side effects include sexual dysfunction, nausea, nervousness, insomnia, and lightheadedness.

The SSRIs most commonly prescribed for Fibromyalgia are Prozac (fluoxetine), Paxil (paroxetine), Effexor (venlafaxine), Zoloft (sertraline), and Cymbalta (duloxetine).

MUSCLE RELAXANTS

Muscle relaxants relieve the pain caused by muscle spasms by inhibiting the spasm. Muscle relaxants are also very sedating, so they help promote sleep. They work by decreasing the transmission of impulses from the spinal cord to skeletal muscles. Possible side effects include drowsiness, dry mouth, constipation, headaches, heart palpitations, abdominal pain, and seizures. Again, avoid alcohol with these medications. Some of the more common muscle relaxants given to fibromyalgia and chronic fatigue syndrome patients are Flexeril (cyclobenzaprine), Soma (carisoprodol), and Robaxin (methocarbamol).

ANTISPASMODICS

These medications are used to treat muscle spasms experienced by patients with conditions such as multiple sclerosis. Antispasmodics work by relaxing muscle spasm, cramping, and tightness as well as lowering the level of the neurotransmitter Substance P, preventing it from signaling the brain to register pain. A person with chronic fatigue syndrome will have a Substance P level three times higher than normal. Possible side effects include hypotension, dry mouth, drowsiness, and nightmares. It is important not to withdraw these medications abruptly because it may precipitate hallucinations or rebound spasticity. The two most common anti-spasmodic medications are baclofen and Zanaflex (tizanidine).

ANTICONVULSANTS

In addition to the treatment of seizures, anticonvulsants are used to treat chronic neuropathic pain (burning and/or electric shock feeling in extremities and nerve irritation). These medications work by smoothing out nerve messages in the brain and causing the brain to respond to the impulses at a steady rate. They should be taken with food. *Do not crush.* The anticonvulsants most commonly used for the treatment of pain are Neurontin (gabapentin), Keppra (levetiracetam), and Lyrica (pregabalin). Lyrica has been approved by the FDA specifically for use for fibromyalgia. Anticonvulsant medication should never be stopped or decreased abruptly because of the risk of developing withdrawal agitation and seizures.

BENZODIAZEPINES

This group of antianxiety drugs, taken at bedtime, is very sedating and helps you to feel calmer and more able to cope with pain. In addition to treating anxiety, benzodiazepines are used for a number of other purposes, including as an anticonvulsant, muscle relaxant, and as a sedative or hypnotic. They are very effective, but there is a risk of abuse or addiction. While some of these drugs are rapidly metabolized and excreted, it is important not to suddenly stop even the ones that linger in the body — especially with those with long half-lives, there is a risk of developing withdrawal anxiety, agitation, and seizures weeks to months after discontinuation. Since benzodiazepines work on the central nervous system, these drugs may be contraindicated if you are taking antihistamines, cold medications, or other OTC and prescription drugs that slow the central nervous system. It is important to AVOID alcohol. Some of the more common benzodiazepines include Klonopin (clonazepam), Valium (diazepam), Xanax (alprazolam), and Ativan (lorazepam).

TRIGGER POINT INJECTIONS

These injections usually contain 1% lidocaine and are injected into fibromyalgia trigger points. When used in combination with physical therapy, the effects usually last three to four weeks.

STATINS

Although this class of drugs is not used for treatment of CFS or fibromyalgia, I include it because it seems that most of the people I know who have these problems also seem to have a problem with high cholesterol levels. Statins are often the treatment of choice for patients with hypercholesterolemia. They work by blocking an enzyme in the liver where cholesterol is made. The statins most often prescribed are Lipitor (atorvastatin), Zocor (simvastatin), Mevacor (lovastatin), Pravachol (pravastatin), Lescol (fluvastatin), and Crestor (rosuvastatin). Blood tests to monitor the functioning of the liver need to be done periodically, as a common side effect is elevated liver enzymes, which may not cause any symptoms for a while, and which may require that the medication must be stopped to prevent damage to the liver.

ALTERNATIVE MEDICINAL THERAPIES

In an effort to relieve their troublesome symptoms, many people with fibromyalgia, chronic fatigue syndrome, and other chronic illnesses have investigated the use of herbs, vitamins, and minerals to ease their pain, gain energy, reduce cognitive difficulties, and improve their general health. Some have reported great success, and it has been my experience that these people don't just jump into any new regimen. They seek out help from experts, read numerous books, and compare alternatives. In other words, they become informed. As you look through this list, remember that the sale of herbal preparations and non-prescription supplements is not regulated by the Food & Drug Administration (FDA), thus the amount of active ingredient in each dose may be highly variable, even if the packaging says otherwise. Here are some of the more popular and favorable treatments:

ST. JOHN'S WORT (hypercicum)

Exactly how this herb works is unclear, but somehow it increases serotonin levels. In the past it was called a "nerve tonic." It helps with mild to moderate depression, helps fight the effects of seasonal affective disorder (SAD), and improves the quality of sleep. St. John's wort has been widely used in Europe for years with success in treating depression. It also relieves uterine cramping and works as an expectorant. When used externally, St. John's wort has antiseptic qualities and is used as a pain reliever for burns, irritations, rheumatism, sciatica, and back pain. It also helps the body fight viral infections. St. John's wort can cause photosensitivity, so avoiding the sun is recommended.

Although St. John's wort is readily available, that does not mean you should use it without some thought. Alone, this herb generally causes no problems when used properly, however there are a number of drugs that can have clinically significant interactions with St. John's wort. *I cannot stress enough the importance of talking to your doctor or pharmacist if you plan on taking this herb*, because if you are already taking an antidepressant, no matter how low the dose, the combination of the two antidepressants could constitute an overdose and may lead to death.

EVENING PRIMROSE OIL

Evening primrose oil (EPO) contains gamma-linolenic acid (GLA), an essential fatty acid that is necessary for healthy cell function. The body is not able to manufacture GLA, so it must be made available in your diet. EPO is especially effective in patients who have become ill after a viral infection with respiratory or GI symptoms. It is not known why EPO works. What is known is that in a great majority of people, it does work and it works well

In his book *New Herb Bible*, Earl Mindell calls evening primrose oil "King's Cure-all," and claims EPO has been used as a painkiller and as an asthma treatment. Studies done in Canada, he says, have shown that EPO helped significantly lower cholesterol levels and blood pressure, relieved symptoms of PMS, alleviated anxiety, and treated schizophrenia. Why, it has even been used to successfully relieve "cradle cap."

MULTIVITAMINS and VITAMIN B

Taking a well-rounded multivitamin and mineral supplement manufactured by a company with integrity will help. If you take B vitamins, I would advise you to take a B-Complex vitamin to assure the right balance of B vitamins.

VITAMIN C (ascorbic acid)

Vitamin C is necessary for collagen formation and tissue repair. Possible side effects, especially with large dosages (greater than 2,000 mg/day) include nausea, vomiting, diarrhea, epigastric burning, acid urine, renal calculi, and renal failure.

Vitamin C is water soluble, meaning the body does not store it, so excess amounts are excreted through urine. Vitamin C *should not be taken with aspirin* because aspirin inhibits the excretion of Vitamin C, which can lead to a toxic build-up.

Vitamin C also aids in the absorption of iron, so if iron supplements are indicated, it is recommended that you take Vitamin C with them.

GINKGO BILOBA

Ginkgo biloba is derived from the leaf of the ginkgo tree. The oldest living tree, the gingko has been studied extensively, yet despite the many studies of its health benefits, nothing has yet been proved conclusively. Its proponents claim ginkgo biloba increases circulation, counteracts the effects of PMS, relieves asthma symptoms, improves memory, benefits MS patients, and cures depression caused by Seasonal Affective Disorder (SAD), among other health conditions.

Caution must be employed when using ginkgo biloba. Its blood thinning properties can cause adverse reactions when taken with medications such as anticoagulants, antihypertensives, antidepressants, and anticonvulsants. You should talk with your doctor or pharmacist before taking ginkgo biloba. It is not to be used by children.

COENZYME Q10 (CoQ10)

Many studies have been done on CoQ10 in an attempt to establish its effectiveness (or lack of effectiveness) in treating many health conditions. The studies, while promising, have not established with a high degree of certainty, just how effective CoQ10 is or can be.

CoQ10 is a proven antioxidant that helps destroy free radicals in the body. Free radicals are thought to accelerate the aging process and can lead to heart disease, cancer, and other health problems.

CoQ10 is a naturally occurring substance found in the body, but is also found in oily fish and organ meats. It is thought to provide energy for the cells and body, and, in partnership with other antioxidants, it is thought to shrink tumors.

CoQ10 is not recommended for use by children.

MALIC ACID and MAGNESIUM

Malic acid is found naturally occurring in the body and can also be obtained from food sources. It plays a large part in the production of energy and has long been used in combination with magnesium to successfully relieve fibromyalgia pain.

Magnesium is a mineral required for a large number of biochemical reactions in the body. Low magnesium levels are known to cause muscle cramping, muscle spasms, and headaches.

Although it takes a few weeks to feel the full benefit of malic acid and magnesium, the pain relief may be significant. When discontinued, pain returns within 48 hours.

VALERIAN

Called the Valium of the 19th century because of its relaxing effect on the body, valerian is used for nervous tension, panic attacks, menstrual cramps, and PMS. One of its drawbacks is that it tastes and smells awful! It may also cause apathy, dizziness, drowsiness, or stomachache.

PASSIONFLOWER (passiflora incarnate)

One of nature's best tranquilizers, passionflower relieves muscle tension and extreme anxiety. It's especially good for nervous insomnia (when you toss and turn all night and are unable to get to sleep). Passionflower also relieves tension headaches and muscle spasms. Do not take during pregnancy.

GLUCOSAMINE

Glucosamine occurs naturally in the body and is a component necessary for the body to synthesize new cartilage. Glucosamine supplements have been used to treat arthritis in animals and humans with good results. It works well to relieve pain and has long-lasting beneficial effects. There are virtually no side effects. Avoid this medication if you are allergic to shellfish or if you are pregnant or nursing. It is safe for use by diabetics.

ACIDOPHILUS ,

Acidophilus is a bacterium (lactobacillus acidophilus) that produces lactic acid, which helps with digestion. If there aren't enough of these "good" bacteria, our bodies can't get the full beneficial nutritional effect from our food, fewer important vitamins will be produced, and the immune system will be rendered less effective. Acidophilus helps alleviate candidiasis and other yeast infections that people with chronic fatigue syndrome and fibromyalgia are prone to.

Acidophilus has been referred to as the "second immune system" because it prevents the growth of disease producing bacteria in the gut.

The aforementioned nutritional supplements are but a few of the more popular supplements used by fibromyalgia and chronic fatigue syndrome patients. Some of the many other supplements available to choose from include:

NADH — a natural coenzyme of vitamin B3, NADH works to increase energy and improve mental clarity.

5-HTP — a compound extracted from griffonia beans taken to improve mood and sleep by helping the body make serotonin.

Conjugated Linoleic Acid (CLA) — helps with weight loss

Flaxseed with borage oil — assists the body's inflammatory response

No matter what regimen you decide to try, *always* check with your doctor and do your research first. Many people have found the free newsletter HEALTHwatch (published by ProHealth) very informative.

The newsletter contains interesting and informative articles written by top experts in the field of fibromyalgia and chronic fatigue syndrome. ProHealth also sells many of the nutritional supplements discussed here. For a free copy of HEALTHwatch, visit www.ImmuneSupport.com online or call 1-800-366-6056.

Remember, there are many alternative remedies available, so be careful and try only one thing at a time so you will recognize the source of possible unwanted side effects. ALWAYS CHECK WITH YOUR DOCTOR before trying something new. Keep a diary similar to the sample daily log found in this book to keep track of both your treatment successes and failures.

11
NUTRITION

You are what you eat.
— Victor Lindlahr, nutritionist

Keep in mind that things are no longer what they once were. Victims of The Thief tend to develop sensitivities or allergies to food products such as milk and milk products, sugars, yeast, caffeine, nuts, corn, wheat, red meat, alcohol, and diet drinks. Frequently the symptoms present as irritable bowel syndrome (IBS), bloating, stomachache, headache, rashes, fatigue, and muscle and/or joint pain.

People with CFS and fibromyalgia need good basic nutrition consisting of the three types of nutrients and foods.

1. Carbohydrates are a principle source of energy for the body but should be taken in moderation. Carbohydrates are found in many food products, especially brown rice, whole-grain pasta, and breads, fresh fruit, and vegetables. A high intake of carbohydrates stimulates insulin production that leads to an excess of insulin in the body. This causes sugar to be released into the muscles and liver where they are converted to fat acids and

118

stored as fat cells. This action prevents the body from using carbohydrates as intended.

2. Proteins: meat, poultry, fish, tofu, and cottage cheese. Eating a high protein diet will ease carbohydrate cravings, give you added energy, and aid in weight loss.

3. Fats: butter, cream, vegetable oil, olive oil. Fats provide an excellent source of energy and are one source of essential fatty acids. Omega-3 fatty acids have anti-inflammatory properties. An Omega-3 or fish oil supplement may be a good idea if you do not eat fish two to three times per week. Fat that is not immediately used as energy for the body is stored in the fat cells under the skin and around internal organs. Excessive fat intake can lead to weight gain and coronary artery disease.

Foods from each of these groups are good to include in your daily diet. One of our support group members recalls back in the 1950s, when exercise guru Jack LaLanne used to admonish everyone to "stay away from the white foods (white bread, white rice, potatoes, sugar), they're poison to you." White foods are bleached and the process of bleaching strips away valuable vitamins and other nutrients.

Another *must* for everyone, and especially the person with The Thief is to drink lots of water. Water serves to hydrate your cells and helps flush out toxins that accumulate in your body.

Of course, common sense also tells us that along with the need for good nutrition is the need to avoid caffeine, tobacco, alcohol, and — I hate to say it — carbonated beverages and chocolate.

The sugar in carbonated beverages brings on an initial spike in energy that soon falls off, causing a roller coaster effect. Besides these energy highs and lows, the 12 to 14 teaspoons of sugar in the average can of soda may lead to yeast problems, especially for person with The Thief.

By burning sugar as its primary source of energy, the body can also become depleted of important vitamins and minerals, especially the B vitamins. Studies have also indicated that carbonated beverages tend to leech phosphorus from bone, which may lead to demineralization of the bones.

As for chocolate, although small quantities of dark chocolate are thought to be good for you, most chocolate candy is very high in fat and calories, and contains small amounts of caffeine.

Being a label reader is important for us all, but especially for the person with The Thief. Sure, it's a pain and takes time, but it's worth the time and effort. I admit freely that I never made it a priority until my husband developed a severe allergy to poultry. It is mind-boggling to realize how many prepared foods list chicken or its byproducts as a part of the ingredients. I picked up a can of baked beans the other day, and, luckily, I read the label. Yep, you guessed it — it contained chicken!

Another ingredient to watch out for is monosodium glutamate (MSG). MSG is a flavor enhancer and preservative that is known to cause headaches, dizziness, and chest pain in susceptible individuals, as well as allergic reactions, which sometimes results in anaphylaxis.

Even beauty products should be scrutinized. Your skin is the largest, most permeable organ in your body, and it absorbs everything that is applied to it. Even some hair dyes can be absorbed through your scalp, eventually working their way into your system to cause a toxic effect.

Along with checking for possible allergens in prepared foods, you should also look for toxins. Yes, that's right, toxins. Poisons. I am speaking specifically of foods containing aspartame. Found mostly in "diet" products such as some sugar-free foods and diet drinks, Aspartame is an excitotoxin that crosses the blood/brain barrier and overstimulates nerve cells. It can cause memory loss along with many other ailments.

No wonder Lisa is always preaching that we should stick to the perimeter of the grocery store when doing our shopping. This is where the natural and unprocessed foods are. Once you start going up and down the aisles, she says, "You're done for." That's where the canned goods and prepared foods with unhealthy preservatives and other "no-nos" are located.

The famous singer/actress, Cher, once did a commercial where she stated, "We care more about what we put in our car than what we put in our bodies!" How true! It's time we cared about ourselves. READ THE LABEL — it could save your life — or at least prevent you from becoming sick.

Along with good nutrition and label reading, everyone, especially the person with The Thief, should practice safe and healthy preparation of foods.

Of course, washing your hands before, during, and after preparing food is a must. Food preparation areas: the refrigerator, cutting boards, and stovetop should be cleaned and disinfected regularly.

Sponges, dishcloths, and towels should be washed regularly as well. Sponges are an ideal breeding ground for bacteria. I wash mine in the dishwasher with the dishes.

Then there's what I refer to as "the dirtiest square inch in the kitchen" — the little cutting wheel on your can opener. Who thinks to keep that clean? It just sits there, quietly attracting bacteria and who knows what else. Just for the heck of it, get yours out now and take a look at it.

I've made a habit of doing something everyone *should* do but usually forget. Wash the tops of cans and boxes before opening. Why? Think about it. All packaged items found in your grocery store have been handled by other people. Why take the chance?

When cooking meat, use two plates — one for the raw meat and the other for the cooked meat. When the meal is over, refrigerate or freeze leftovers within two hours and store them in the smallest covered container possible. I find those zip-lock plastic bags invaluable for storing leftovers. It's also a good idea to label and date each item. And, of course, when it comes to leftovers, it's always safest to stick to the old adage, "When in doubt, throw it out."

When preparing fresh foods, instead of boiling them to death and losing all the goodness they have to offer, try using a steamer. It takes less energy to cook, doesn't heat up the kitchen as much, and foods retain more of their nutritional value.

We wanted to include here a few recipes from a cookbook put together by our support group. We hope you'll try them and enjoy them.

NO NAME CHICKEN DISH

Mix ¼ cup flour with ⅔ cup water, making sure there are no lumps.

Add 2 tsp granulated (not cubed) chicken bouillon and 1 Tbsp Butter Buds

Pour the mixture into a saucepan and heat.

Stir or whisk until mixture thickens and add 1 more cup water. Continue stirring and heating until the mixture is thick and not lumpy. Remove from heat.

To the above mixture add:

2 cooked and sliced or diced carrots, 1 box frozen cauliflower, the meat of three cooked chicken thighs and ½ cup frozen peas. (The heat of the dish will be enough to warm up and "defrost" the peas.)

Reheat and serve over toast or crackers.

Optional: for a special treat I sometimes add some cooked shrimp

JELL-O PARFAIT

Make Jell-o gelatin in the flavor of your choice according to package directions.

When mixture is thick but not quite jelled, add ⅔ cup non-fat dry milk and whip with electric mixer for several minutes, making sure *all* of the milk has blended in. Mixture will increase *significantly* (at least 3-4 times) in volume.

Put mixture back in refrigerator until it jells completely. You will have a light, airy, chiffon-like dessert.

CAULIFLOWER NUGGETS

¾ cup plain or seasoned bread crumbs

⅓ cup grated Parmesan/Romano cheese

2 egg whites (I use powdered egg whites)

1 tsp water

Cauliflower florets (fresh, not frozen)

PAM butter flavored spray oil

Combine the breadcrumbs and grated cheese in a plastic zip-lock bag. Mix well.

Stir the egg whites and water together. Coat cauliflower florets with the egg white mixture and place them in the plastic bag with bread-crumbs and cheese. Shake well to coat. Place the florets on a cookie sheet, spray with PAM, and bake at 350 degrees for about 20 minutes or until golden brown.

Serve with a small bowl of spaghetti sauce or ranch dressing for dipping if desired.

NO PEEK STEW

2 lb stew beef

1 package onion soup mix

1 can mushrooms, drained

1 can golden mushroom soup

1 cup ginger ale

Mix all ingredients together, cover, and bake at 350 degrees for 2 hours.

This is so simple because there is no need to brown the meat and the aroma of the meal as it bakes is awesome. A little more ginger ale may be added if desired as well as a few potatoes and carrots.

And now — for my MOST favorite recipe of all:

LISA'S F.I.N.E. MEAL

F - ast

I - nteresting

N - utritious

E - asy

Go to your refrigerator. Look at all the foil wrapped packages and Tupperware containing something lumpy, greenish/grayish, and unidentifiable inside. Close the refrigerator door and vow NEVER to open it again until you have conned someone else into cleaning it out.

Go to your telephone and press the speed dial for the meal of your choice (chicken, pizza, subs, Chinese, or whatever).

Order your supper to be delivered. (Since you're by now on a first name basis with the delivery person, don't forget to ask how he or she and the family are doing.)

After following this recipe you will be sitting down to eat a delicious, nutritious, stress-free meal (with no dishes to wash) within a half hour.

In summary:

1. BECOME A LABEL READER.
2. Prepare your food in a sanitary manner.
3. Make healthy food choices, even if you use the takeout method.

Americans tend to be overweight because of poor nutritional habits. We have become a fast food, high carbohydrate society. The key to good health, more energy, and less fatigue is to make healthier food choices so your body can work efficiently, like it is meant to.

12
SLEEP

How short the night to him that sleeps.
— Unknown

Okay, we all know that we need sleep. But *why* do we need sleep? Strictly speaking, from my perspective as one who has a few sleep problems, I need sleep because it feels good and I need to feel good. For most people, I suppose they sleep because they have to.

Good, restorative sleep gives your body a chance to slow down, take a deep breath, and restore itself. Muscles, cells, and organs are given the opportunity to repair while the brain slows down and "rests" awhile.

When awake and alert, your brain generates fast brain waves, and when you sleep the brain waves slow down. The slower the brain wave, the deeper the sleep, which makes a person in this state more difficult to awaken.

What happens while you are asleep? First, you will generally be lying down. (Although the male members of my husband's family could fall asleep on a bed of nails in the middle of a hurricane!) Usually, you are completely relaxed. Breathing and heart rate are slowed. The only difference between being asleep and being unconscious or comatose is that you can't arouse an unconscious person; whereas strong stimuli can awaken a sleeping person.

During a night's sleep cycle two types of sleep are experienced: REM (rapid eye movement) and non-REM (non-rapid eye movement) sleep. You must experience both types in order to get a restful night's sleep. It's during the REM stage that you dream. You can tell when a person (or animal) is in the REM stage of sleep because their body twitches and their eyes move rapidly back and forth.

During REM sleep your body is almost completely paralyzed, except for the diaphragm and other muscles required for breathing. If you wake a person during REM sleep they can usually vividly recall their dreams. Dreams usually last from five to thirty minutes. A person in non-REM sleep is not dreaming.

You may wonder why we dream. Electrical impulses are sent randomly through the brain about every 90 minutes during sleep. The brain tries but can't make sense of these impulses. How our brain "sees" these random impulses creates dreams that may be able to tell us something about ourselves (like the Rorschach ink blots in psychological testing).

Although we cannot control our dreams, we know that dreams usually involve ourselves, and most relate to something that has happened recently. We may be trying to work out some deep-seated problem, wishes, fears, or anxiety via our dreams.

What happens when you don't get enough restorative sleep? Missing one night of sleep is not fatal. If you miss one night of sleep, the next day you may be either irritable or completely wired. After two nights without sleep, things get worse. Concentration is difficult. You make mistakes and may feel apathetic. After three nights without sleep you are unable to think coherently and you may begin to hallucinate and lose your grasp on reality. Laboratory rats that have been forced to stay continuously awake will soon die.

Even if you manage to get a few hours sleep each night, you may still experience problems. Growth hormones and substances important to the immune system are secreted during sleep, which means you can become susceptible to disease. A child's growth can be stunted if they don't get proper amounts of restorative sleep.

The amount of sleep needed varies by individual and changes with age. Generally speaking, the average person needs seven to nine hours of good, restorative sleep per night. The younger you are the more sleep you need. An infant needs twenty or more hours of sleep per day. A toddler needs about twelve hours, pre-teens need about ten hours, and adults can usually get by with seven to nine hours of sleep each night.

Are you having trouble sleeping? Try one or more of these ideas:

- No caffeine, tobacco or other stimulants after 4:00 p.m.
- Exercise regularly, but not right before bedtime.
- Avoid alcohol before bedtime.

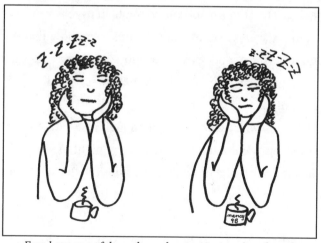

Ever have one of those days when you just can't wake up?

- Establish good sleep hygiene. Go to bed and get up the same time every day, even on weekends.
- Take a long, warm, relaxing bath. Adding Epsom salts works well to soothe sore muscles.
- Drink a glass of warm milk.
- Sleep in a comfortable room with plenty of ventilation.
- Use a good, firm mattress.
- Avoid naps.
- Get rid of your illuminated clock.
- Drink a cup of herbal tea.
- Try sleeping on your back.
- Ask your bed partner to give you a massage.
- If after 20 minutes you aren't asleep, get up and do something relaxing until you feel sleepy.
- Do not "sleep in."
- Play tricks on yourself, such as pretending you want to stay awake.
- Listen to soothing music.
- If you find your body tensing up, do the relaxation exercise discussed in Chapter 9, Alternative Therapies.
- Visualize — something pleasant, something boring, whatever works for you.
- Do *not* watch TV in bed.
- Use you bedroom for sleep and sex only. NO TV, NO COMPUTER, NO DISTRACTIONS.
- Have some sort of white noise (such as a fan) in the background.
- See how high you can count or try to name all 50 states and their capitals.

- Get up earlier in the morning.
- Review your medications with your doctor, as some medications can interfere with sleep.
- Ask your doctor to order a sleep study.

A chapter about sleep would not be complete without a discussion about Restless Legs Syndrome (RLS). RLS is *finally* being recognized and accepted as a neurological condition affecting up to eight percent of people in the United States. To those of you lucky enough to *not* have restless legs let me describe what it's like. RLS makes you feel as if your legs are filled to overflowing with ants crawling around inside your skin. The only relief comes from moving your legs. It usually occurs only in the legs and at night, however, some people (like me) experience the symptoms 24/7/365 in the legs *and* the arms.

Typically the symptoms are present when the person is at rest and are relieved by movement. Your bed partner may tell you that you jerk your legs frequently during the night. You wake up feeling tired and as if you were hit by a Mack truck. Approximately eighty percent of people with RLS also experience Periodic Limb Movement Disorder (PLMD), which causes partial arousals that disrupt sleep.

As with The Thief, no definite cause is known and there is no definitive cure for RLS. Some research points to it being a genetic disorder. Or, it may be secondary to pregnancy or another condition. With secondary RLS, symptoms worsen while the primary condition exists and goes away when the primary condition resolves. Other secondary causes of RLS may be anemia, low blood levels of iron, kidney failure, and peripheral neuropathy. It has recently been discovered that there is a correlation between RLS and the symptoms of attention deficit disorder. And, of course, there is the old standby cause — idiopathic, meaning you have it because you have it and no one can explain why.

I experienced symptoms of RLS off and on throughout my life until I met The Thief and my RLS symptoms increased in frequency and severity. It was only after my doctor ordered a sleep study that my problem was recognized and I received treatment. I am happy to say that I now have the symptoms under control *if* I take my medication on time. Mind you, while the symptoms are under control, the condition *is not cured.*

Treatment for RLS is based upon careful analysis of your problem and how to achieve the desired goal with the fewest problems. For example, if pregnancy seems to be the cause, then it is likely the RLS will go away after the birth of the baby. If anemia appears to be the cause, your doctor may want to supplement your diet with iron, Vitamin B-12, or folate. When taking iron supplements you should have your serum ferritin level checked as often as your doctor recommends.

Some medications may cause RLS symptoms to worsen. If this is the case, work with your doctor and pharmacist to find an acceptable alternative. A healthy, well-balanced diet and good sleep hygiene are a must. Avoiding caffeine and alcohol can also help lessen the severity of RLS.

Some activities that may also help relieve symptoms include walking, stretching, taking a hot or cool bath, massaging the affected limb(s), hot or cold packs, or distracting yourself by getting involved in a game, book, or playing on the computer. Unfortunately, I have found that only some of these work for me, and if they do, it's only for a short time and then the symptoms return.

There are currently only two FDA approved drugs for RLS, but some medications used for other conditions can also be quite effective. These medications fall into four classes:

Dopaminergic agents are the first line of pharmacological treatment. Dopaminergic-receptor agonists add dopamine to your system. When taking a dopaminergic, you should start out with a very low dose, gradually increasing the dose as prescribed by your health care provider. Some dopaminergics are Mirapex (pramipexole), Requip (ropinirole), Permax (pergolide — was withdrawn from the U.S. market in 2007), and Sinemet (carbidopa/levodopa). You may notice that while these drugs are also used to treat Parkinson's disease, RLS is *not* related to Parkinson's disease. It is important also to be aware that if you use any of the dopamine agonists, the chance of augmentation occurring is significant. Augmentation is when a drug works and relief is obtained but symptoms may begin to occur earlier in the day and increase in intensity and frequency. If augmentation occurs, let your doctor know so that you can be started on another medication.

Sedatives are the most effective method of alleviating RLS symptoms. They are usually given at night along with a dopaminergic for best results. Klonopin (clonazepam) is the sedative most commonly used for this purpose but has significant side effects including constipation, falls, and excessive sleepiness.

Opioid prescription pain-relievers like Darvon or Darvocet (propoxyphene), Dolophine (methadone), Percocet (oxycodone), Ultram (tramadol), and Vicodin (hydrocodone) are as effective for use in RLS as sedatives but because of the potential for abuse, doctors generally don't like to prescribe them.

You *must* have your condition well documented by your health care provider. And although it is not diagnostic of RLS, a sleep study offers proof and validation of your condition so that you do not appear to be a drug seeker.

Anticonvulsants work for some patients with RLS symptoms that are also associated with pain syndromes. Neurontin (gabapentin) is the medication of choice in this case.

The following medications should be *AVOIDED* if you have RLS:

Anti-nausea medications such as Benadryl (diphenhydramine), Antivert or Bonine (meclizine), Atarax or Vistaril (hydroxyzine), Compazine (prochlorperazine), Phenergan (promethazine), Thorazine (chlorpromazine), Tigan (trimethobenzamide), Trilafon (perphenazine), and Reglan (metoclopramide).

Use instead: Kytril (granisetron) or Zofran (ondansetron).

Anti-psychotic medications such as Haldol (haloperidol), Loxitane (loxapine), Mellaril (thioridazine), Navane (thiothixene), Prolixin (fluphenazine), Risperdal (risperidone), Serentil (mesoridazine), Stelazine (trifluoperazine), Thorazine (chlorpromazine), and Vesprin (triflupromazine).

Instead, use the following "atypical neuroleptic drugs" WITH CAUTION: Clozaril (clozapine), Seroquel (quetiapine), or Zyprexa (olanzapine).

Antidepressant medications can cause significant worsening of symptoms in many patients with RLS. Tricyclics such as Elavil (amitriptyline), Pamelor (nortriptyline), Asendin (amoxapine), and Limbitrol (amitriptyline-chlordiazepoxide) and the serotonin reuptake inhibitors (SSRIs) Celexa (citalopram), Serzone (nefazodone), Zoloft (sertraline), Paxil (paroxetine), and Prozac (fluoxetine). Wellbutrin (bupropion), a dopamine-active antidepressant may prove to be effective when others are not.

The health care consumer with RLS must also be careful with over-the-counter medications. Beware of all antihistamines, especially Benadryl and OTC or prescription combination cough-cold-sinus preparations like Actifed, Comtrex, Contact, Dimetapp, Triaminic, TheraFlu, Vick's cough syrup, Tylenol PM, Excedrin PM, and Bayer PM. These products provide excellent symptom relief for allergies or colds *if* you do not have RLS.

For those of you in the health care field, I can't say this strongly enough — restraining a patient with RLS should be avoided at all costs! RLS is a neurological disorder that causes an *irresistible* urge to move and keep moving the limbs. To use restraints on a person with RLS would be extremely cruel. It's better to let the patient continue with his/her treatment of choice and/or give their prescribed RLS/PLMD medications.

There is certainly more information available, especially about medications, but I have chosen to touch on the most common ones here. To learn more, talk with your doctor, consult with a sleep specialist, and join a support group. They can all be valuable sources of information and are more than willing to share their knowledge and experience with you.

Finally, I would be remiss if I did not mention the Restless Legs Syndrome Foundation. As someone with RLS/PLMD (plus yet another sleep disorder, REM behavior disorder) I have found the foundation's publications invaluable, and would like to offer a hearty, "Thank You" for their work providing education about RLS. This wonderful organization presents cutting-edge information on their website and in their quarterly magazine, "Night Walkers." Contact the RLS Foundation at 1610 14th St. NW, Suite 300, Rochester, MN 55901, phone 507-287-6465, or on the web at www.rls.org.

I can find humor in nearly every aspect of my illness but I can find no humor in having RLS.

13
EXERCISE

The pain passes but the beauty remains.
— Renoir

Exercise programs work for some but should be approached cautiously, sensibly, and with the full knowledge and approval of your primary physician or rheumatologist. Generally speaking, people with

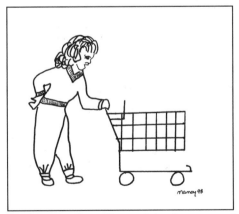

You know you have fibromyalgia when you need a shopping cart even when you're just window-shopping.

fibromyalgia will benefit from exercise, while for people with chronic fatigue syndrome it may put them over the edge and bring on a flare.

Exercise such as water aerobics and walking have proved beneficial for some people, but again, everything in moderation. Before beginning an exercise program, I think it's important that you first do some research to determine which form of exercise is best for you. Start with the simplest of routines. Set *reasonable* goals for yourself. Ask yourself, what do you (realistically) want to achieve? How soon do you want to achieve it?

The least expensive, easiest, and most readily available form of exercise is walking, but *do not* go out and walk several miles on your first outing. If you begin by overexerting, your exercise program is doomed from the start and you will most likely give up exercise forever. It may take a year to reach your goals, but that's okay. Alter your goals to accommodate your illness.

Trying to maintain pre-illness fitness goals is not realistic and isn't fair to you or your body. You will tire faster, your pain will increase, and your self-esteem will suffer. Start out slowly. Walk ten minutes a day three or four days a week, then gradually increase your time and distance.

Keep a fitness diary, recording your distance, time, weather conditions, and how you feel after walking. Make sure to record your activities daily to help track your progress and attain your goals. Keep your doctor informed of your accomplishments.

Use your walking time to relax your mind and spirit. Entertain yourself by honing your observations skills; watch for wildlife and identify different birds and plants. Or do a good deed as a friend of mine does and bring a plastic bag along to pick up trash from the side of the road as you walk.

Dress comfortably for the weather, and it wouldn't hurt to carry a walking stick. Wear light or brightly colored clothing so that you are more visible to drivers.

It's also a good idea to leave a note or let someone know where you are going and when you expect to be back.

You will find after a time that you'll miss your daily walk if for some reason you're not able to get out. When the weather is inhospitable, many walkers seek the controlled climate of their local shopping mall. A treadmill can be a valuable piece of equipment and a good investment for when you're unable to get outside.

Other tricks you can employ to get your walking in may be as simple as parking farther away from the store or mall or using the stairs rather than elevators or escalators.

If walking causes pain or makes you feel unwell, curtail your walking program for a while and let your doctor know.

Water aerobics is another excellent form of exercise. The temperature of the water should be approximately 90 degrees for maximum comfort. Sign up for a class or just walk around the shallow end of the pool with your arms under the water for ease of movement. Many community pools or YMCA pools can be used by the general public. Or join a fitness gym where they will likely have staff on hand to lend assistance if needed.

My favorite exercise is my stationary bike. I can get on it in the privacy of my own home, wear old sweatpants, turn on the TV or radio, or get a favorite book and pedal away to my heart's content. If I want fresh air I just open a door or window.

Besides strengthening your body and improving your health, exercising regularly helps with weight control. Less weight equals decreased pain and decreased risk of diabetes and heart disease. Most people with

CFS or FM gain an average of fifty pounds or more when they become ill.

Pain, poor sleep, mitral valve prolapse, TMJ, irritable bowel, fibro-fog, etc., *and* a fifty-pound weight gain to boot! Sometimes life just isn't fair!

14
STRESS

Adopting the right attitude can convert a negative
stress into a positive one.
— Dr. Hans Selye

Stress can be good — celebrating a wedding or a baptism, or winning the lottery. Stress can be bad — the death of a loved one or a failing relationship. Your body does not differentiate between good or bad stress. Good or bad, stress is stress and your body *reacts* the same way regardless.

When your body reacts to stress, certain physical phenomena occur in order to help you handle that stress. To better understand what happens, imagine the following scenario: it's a bright, sunny, summer day. You are on a delightful walk in the woods. You're walking happily along, whistling a merry tune. All is right with your world when suddenly you stop in your tracks! Right in front of you is the biggest, ugliest, fiercest, HUNGRIEST Tyrannosaurus Rex you have ever seen! (Congratulations on your wonderful imagination.)

Now let's freeze-frame that image and examine what is happening to your body and why, as the "fight or flight" response is activated and you run for your life.

- All the blood vessels to the periphery of your body become dilated (larger) so blood can reach your muscles faster, supplying the boost of energy needed to get away from that nasty dinosaur. At the same time, blood vessels to your gut constrict (become smaller), moving blood away from your gut where it is not needed at the moment, to the tissues that do need it.

- Your heart rate increases in order to pump blood faster.

- Your respiratory (breathing) rate increases, taking in more oxygen and expelling carbon dioxide at a faster rate.

- The pupils of your eyes dilate to allow more light in, sharpening your vision. When fleeing from danger you need to see where you are going and, if you have to fight, you want to be able to connect.

Finally, you reach safety and all body systems return to normal. WHEW!!! Your body has had quite a workout! All systems *adapted* to resist that stressful encounter and to preserve your life. These adaptations, though, come with a price — that is a decrease in your ability to resist illness.

Stress can also trigger a desire to eat more food than you need (especially sugar) and also causes a release of adrenalin. Adrenalin is a hormone produced by the adrenals, small glands located on top of the kidneys. Part of the endocrine system, their main job is the secretion of adrenalin. Adrenalin is released in higher levels during times of stress to help the body cope. However, adrenalin release *also* stresses your body and can trigger a flare of your symptoms. Excess adrenalin release can also cause panic attacks. Low adrenal function is manifested by symptoms of weakness and dehydration.

As you go through life you experience many changes — some good, some bad. These changes are referred to by some psychologists as Life Change Units (LCUs). Each LCU brings with it a degree of stress, which you have learned requires an expenditure of energy. In order to survive, your body *must* respond and adapt to stress.

Researchers have compiled a list of Life Change Units, giving each life change a number value. The number of life changes experienced over a six-month to one-year period can indicate whether you may develop a serious illness and how seriously you are affected by it. You can see how stress affects your body and how it correlates with your illness.

Don't get excited or stressed now, but it's time for a quick quiz. We are not grading you. In fact, *you* will be grading yourself. Get a piece of paper and a pencil or calculator and let's start adding up your score to see if you need to prepare for what lies ahead for you — health-wise that is.

In 1967, Dr. Thomas H. Holmes and Dr. Richard H. Rahe developed the Social Readjustment Rating Scale to gauge the impact of stress on health. Below is the rescaled, updated version of Rahe and Miller's Recent Life Changes Questionnaire (1997) with its revised Life Change Units. Your final score indicates how the life changes you experience impact your health. The incidence of illness in relation to the number of life change units over a six-month to one-year period is an indicator of the seriousness of illness you may experience. The higher the number of LCUs, the higher your risk of developing serious illness.

RECENT LIFE CHANGES QUESTIONNAIRE

Life Event	Men	Women
Death of a son or daughter	135	103
Death of a spouse	122	113
Death of a brother or sister	111	87
Death of a parent	105	90
Divorce	102	85
Death of a family member	96	78
Fired from work	85	69
Separation from spouse due to marital problems	79	70
Major illness or injury	79	64
Being held in jail	78	71
Pregnancy	74	55
Miscarriage or abortion	74	51
Death of a close friend	73	64
Laid off from work	73	59
Birth of a child	71	56
Adopting a child	71	54
Major business adjustment	67	47
Decrease in income	66	49
Parents divorce	63	52
A relative moving in with you	62	53
Foreclosure on a mortgage or loan	62	51
Investment and/or credit difficulties	62	46
Marital reconciliation	61	48
Major change in health or behavior of family member	58	50
Change in arguments with spouse	55	41
Retirement	54	48
Major decision regarding your immediate future	54	46
Separation from spouse due to work	53	54
An accident	53	38
Parental remarriage	52	45
Change in residence to a different town, city, state	52	39
Change to a new type of work	51	50
"Falling out" of a close, personal relationship	50	41
Marriage	50	50
Spouse changes at work	50	38
Child leaving home	48	38
Birth of a grandchild	48	34
Engagement to marry	47	42
Moderate illness	37	35
Loss or damage of personal property	47	35
Sexual difficulties	44	44
Getting demoted at work	44	39

Life Event	Men	Women
Major change in living conditions	44	37
Increase in income	43	30
Relationship problems	42	34
Trouble with in-laws	41	33
Beginning or ending school or college	40	35
Making a major purchase	40	33
New, close personal relationship	39	33
Outstanding personal achievement	38	33
Troubles with co-workers at work	37	32
Change in school or college	37	31
Change in work hours or conditions	36	32
Trouble with workers whom you supervise	35	34
Getting a transfer at work	33	31
Getting a promotion at work	33	29
Change in religious beliefs	31	27
Christmas	30	25
Having more responsibilities at work	29	29
Troubles with your boss at work	29	29
Major change in usual type or amount of recreation	29	29
General work troubles	29	27
Change in social activities	29	24
Major change in eating habits	29	23
Major change in sleeping habits	28	23
Change in family get-togethers	28	20
Change in personal habits	27	24
Major dental work	27	23
Change of residence in same town, city	27	21
Change in political beliefs	26	21
Vacation	26	20
Having fewer responsibilities at work	22	21
Making a moderate purchase	22	18
Change in church activities	21	20
Minor violation of the law	20	18
Correspondence course to help you in your work	19	16

Add up the total number of life change units you have experienced over the last six to twelve months. If your total exceeds 300 after six months or 500 points after a year, you are at high risk for experiencing serious health problems.

What is your score? I stopped adding when mine reached 465. Taking all of this into consideration, it's no wonder we get sick. It is a well-known theory in physics that for every *action*, there is an equal and opposite *reaction*. Look again at the list of "actions" that you have experienced. The compulsory reactions have got to manifest themselves somewhere. And they do — in the health of your body.

So then the question becomes how can I reduce this stress and stay healthy? One important part of the process is to continue to do all of the things we talked about so far in the book: eat well, exercise, get a good night's sleep, take your medications, and keep your doctor informed about what is going on in your life. We'll cover one additional aspect, spirituality, in the next chapter.

But this still leaves the question about what to do with all the events that are causing the stress. Here is a suggestion that works for me.

When you face multiple problems and you think everything needs to be fixed right away, just STOP. Decide which problem seems most important and focus on that first. Solve one problem before moving on to the next. Chances are that by the time the third problem is "fixed," all the others will have resolved themselves or will no longer seem as problematic. Only the Ten Commandants are written in stone. Everything else is subject to change.

The following story illustrates how problem solving and learning to take care of yourself can work hand-in-hand.

BOB

Bob never had any serious illness as a child. Oh, he had the usual childhood illnesses like measles, mumps, coughs and colds, but nothing out of the ordinary.

Bob was a typical boy growing up, leading a very active life, playing sports, and holding down many different part-time jobs to earn spending money. He mowed lawns, shoveled snow, and delivered papers.

Bob had lots of friends to hang out with and was a fun-loving, mischievous, hell-raising kid who loved to tease the girls. He had a big heart and a generous spirit. He never caused anyone any kind of pain.

As a young man, Bob moved from job to job, gaining valuable experience in many different professions while developing a strong work ethic and learning to adapt to any given situation. A couple of hitches in the armed services did much to fine-tune his outlook and turned him into a mature, responsible, and serious citizen. He exhibited the traits of your typical Type-A personality. He felt the need to accomplish many things at once and accomplish it all to perfection. Nothing less would do.

When he reached his early fifties, Bob began to experience some pain, achiness, and sleeplessness. He put his adaptive skills to use and became adept at ignoring his symptoms until there finally came a point he could no longer ignore them. The pain became worse. He was so exhausted he could barely function. A good night's sleep was a distant memory. He started forgetting things. Bob finally had to admit to himself that this was more than "just getting old" and he began to worry. Could this be the beginning of Alzheimer's? That's all I need, he thought. Might as well get it over with and find out for sure.

Bob went to his doctor who proceeded to do all the standard tests. Everything came back normal. Now what? If it's not Alzheimer's, then what is it? His doctor suggested some of the catchall diagnoses — polymyalgia, rheumatism, etc. But his doctor could give no definitive diagnosis.

Bob went home, continued with his own treatment plan, and turned to his computer. After a lot of research, Bob found his own diagnosis. In fact, it felt like he was reading about someone else living his life.

Bob discovered he had fibromyalgia. He went back to his doctor, presented him with his findings, and the two began working together to try to find an acceptable solution to the problems fibromyalgia presented.

Bob found some relief, enough to allow him to function. He accepts his diagnosis stoically, looking at it as just another hurdle life has thrown at him. He remains an engaging, outgoing personality, striving for perfection. *But,* the most important thing he's learned is to temper his expectations of himself and he now approaches his life and career with common sense.

Bob learned a valuable life lesson — he takes care of himself and does only what he feels he can do without causing more pain. He's done this without sacrificing a thing, and in doing so has become a valued member of his community and his support group.

Another lesson that can be very hard to learn is to let someone else help. I don't know if you've noticed, but there has been a common theme that has shown up in all of the stories in the book — the people have all tried to accomplish many things and they have felt they needed to accomplish them on their own. Maybe they thought other people were unable to do the work. Maybe they wanted to spare other people bad feelings. What happened in the end was that they couldn't do everything that they wanted to do. If you want to reduce your stress, you need to learn that lesson, too.

Call on others for help. There's an old saying that joy shared is doubled and pain shared is cut in half. Letting someone help with your many tasks is a way to get them done. You don't have to do everything yourself. Realizing that the things that need to be done don't need to be done by *you* will go a long way toward relieving your stress. There is more about this idea in the next chapter.

15
SPIRITUALITY AND THE THIEF

A day hemmed in prayer will not soon unravel.
— Unknown

Some people may feel uncomfortable with this subject; others may feel something is missing if we don't mention it. Spiritual faith is an area we feel is too often overlooked and feel strongly that it has a rightful place in this book.

As renaissance poet and clergyman, John Donne, wrote in his meditations, "No man is an island." People need people. From the moment of your birth until your last breath on earth, people will enter and exit your life, each one leaving a mark on you whether you are aware of it or not.

You may not believe in the same God I believe in, or you may express your faith differently, or you may not believe in God at all. The important message is not a particular belief, but the idea that there is an overriding spirit in this world that will help you deal with your illness. I know this spirit as the God represented in the Holy Bible and the fellowship in my church. You may also find it in God. You may find it in

148

nature. You may find it in your fellowship with others. What is important is that you find it and use it to help you live well with your disease. I will share my belief here and ask you to consider trying it if your current path is not bringing you the spiritual comfort you need.

I am keenly aware of this one fact. Are you ready? I thank God for having The Thief in my life. Yes, I'll say it again, "Thank you, God!" For if I did not have this terrible, painful, exasperating, mystifying, expensive, horrible illness, I would not have met and come to know and love some of the most wonderful, loving, caring people in the world — people I am *honored* to call my friends — the people in my support group.

GOD WORKS IN MYSTERIOUS WAYS
HIS WONDERS TO PERFORM

Every life has a purpose — a reason for being. There are many paths you may take to lead you to that purpose and you must make many decisions and choices along the way. Some will be good. Some will be bad. But even when you make a bad decision, you still have a chance to make it good. You can turn a bad choice into something positive. I firmly believe that you learn more from your failures than you do from your successes.

We must learn to take control of our lives and not let the pain we feel control us. We must have faith. Ask for a daily blessing. God will heal you. He is with you. He is the way. He is the truth. He is the light.

You could give up and spend your life asking, "Why me? Why did this happen to me?" That's a bad choice. It happened and there is nothing left for you to do but to accept it. I know. I made the wrong choice. I was once filled with doom and gloom and kept thinking and asking, "Why me?" Not that I necessarily wanted it to be someone else, but still, "Why me?" I failed to realize and remember that God has a plan for each and every one of us. Now, mind you, His plan and my plan may not be the same — but, let's face it, He's the boss. It's up to me to adjust, not Him. So now instead of asking, "Why me?" I ask, "Why *not* me?"

By accepting God's plan for me, I have been able to help myself and others. Now that I have "God Power," I no longer waste my time in self-pity. I am instead, "wising my time."

When I say I'm "wising my time", I mean that my time is now spent helping others to help themselves. Helping others to regain their sense of direction and self worth; helping others to learn to cope and accept, to adjust to their illness, and enable them to live their lives to the fullest, despite this horrible illness. And, wonder of wonders, by doing that I am also helping myself.

GOD WORKS IN MYSTERIOUS WAYS
HIS WONDERS TO PERFORM

Lauren's story reflects how anger and frustration can lead you back to God for strength and comfort, and help you make something positive of a very difficult situation.

LAUREN

If you didn't know the definition of "Yuppie," all you would need to do is look at Lauren. Attractive, young, active, and intelligent, Lauren wore designer clothes and drank Perrier. Her life was on an upward spiral. She was well on her way to earning her Master's degree. A wonderful, loving, handsome "Mr. Right" had entered her life, and they decided to marry. She had a great job with lots of responsibility and earned a phenomenal salary. She had a new home and was soon expecting a baby. Life was great!

Then one day a careless driver crossed her path and changed her life. Lauren was five months pregnant at the time and the automobile accident left her requiring multiple surgeries for relentless, agonizing back pain. Because she was pregnant Lauren was unable to have diagnostic x-rays or MRIs at the time. When back surgery was finally performed, it was not successful in relieving her pain. And she had CFS.

It's not unusual for people to pinpoint an accident or other trauma as the start of their CFS symptoms. It was formerly thought that such an incident may be the precipitating factor in developing CFS. However, now that we suspect that CFS may be caused by a virus, it is accepted as a possibility that a traumatic physical or emotional event can somehow awaken a dormant virus, bringing about the misery of CFS.

It wasn't long before Lauren was no longer able to function well at her job. She'd call in sick, or, if she made it to work, she had to leave early, unable to bear her pain.

Pain often left her bedridden, and she had a new baby to care for. Her memory and cognition were so bad she would get lost in her own home. Because of this Lauren was forced to abandon her hopes of completing her degree.

Then Lauren's plans and dreams of having more children were dashed when she had to undergo an emergency hysterectomy, causing more physical and emotional stress. Lauren managed to hide her feelings of loss and disappointment and get on with her life. She was a determined woman, and, with the help of a very supportive husband, she learned how to cope.

She had a lot of anger and resentment, though. She felt like a victim. "Why me?" she asked. "Why can't I have what I once had? What I planned for? I EARNED it!" She was very angry. She felt God had deserted her and she resented that.

The role of being a victim wasn't comfortable, though, so she gave up the role and became emotionally stronger day by day. She eventually accepted her illness and began looking for a way to help others with the same problems to understand and accept their condition. She met Sophia and Helen, helped start a support group, and went on to become very active in the group's activities. Taking her "job" as support group leader to heart, Lauren educated herself and others about her illness.

Lauren had always been a religious person and now she opened the door to her heart and soul. She invited God back in, realizing that, without knowing it, she was following His path. The path He set for her. She knew that God wanted her to be His tool to provide others the help they needed and His reward was bringing Helen, Sophia, and many other wonderful people into her life. She now feels blessed to have this horrible illness. That may sound trite — even stupid, but Lauren swears it's the truth. And I know it's true, because that's how I feel, too.

Remember, God has a plan for each and every one of us. He knows the plan He has for *you*. Be patient — things happen in His time, not yours. Have faith that He will not give you more of a burden than you can bear. I know sometimes it may feel you cannot bear it, but trust me — and yourself. You can do this. Why *not* you?

GOD WORKS IN MYSTERIOUS WAYS
HIS WONDERS TO PERFORM

16
PSYCHOLOGICAL
ASPECTS OF THE THIEF

Dreaming allows each and every one of us to be quietly
and safely insane every night of our lives
— William Demen

This is an illness that affects *every* area of your life. You must understand that you will be affected physically, emotionally, socially,
financially, and sexually. The five stages of grief apply not only in
reaction to a death, but can also apply to any critical or chronic situation.
You must grieve well and successfully if you are to come to realistic
terms with your condition.

The stages of grief are:

Denial. In an effort to try to convince yourself, you will deny that
you have the illness — that someone screwed up somewhere. It's not
possible to have "that" happen to me. The diagnosis is wrong, absolutely
bogus. You will not discuss the subject and your attitude may be "there's
nothing wrong, nothing at all."

Anger. After a length of time (anywhere from one hour to years later) you realize that you *do* indeed have the illness, and boy, are you ANGRY ! You make no effort to hold your anger in. This stage is quite difficult for your family and friends, especially when they try to help. Words and objects may fly as fits of anger are expressed.

Bargaining. At this point you "sort of" accept the inevitable, or you may be willing to accept it. But only if you can live long enough to see your son graduate from college or until your grandchild is born, or some other long awaited event occurs.

Depression. All pretenses and emotion are gone. The weight of the world is upon you as you face the losses and inevitable future (or lack of it) that awaits you. You become locked in your own black world and refuse to allow anyone in. The length of time spent in this stage, as in all other stages, varies.

Acceptance. In this, the last stage, your family and friends begin to see the change in you. You have finally found a way to move forward and you know it's going to be okay. All the doubt, anger, and depression are gone and you have finally accepted the inevitable.

These stages are universal and we mention them so that you will know them when you see them and recognize them in yourself or a loved one. And we want to let you know that you are not alone. What you are experiencing is normal and expected. The goal is to reach stage five — that of acceptance of your condition and current situation. You will feel better physically and emotionally at this point. You will not, however, reach that stage until you have at least briefly gone through the preceding four stages. Some people get stuck in one stage and never move forward. Some go back and forth through the stages before reaching acceptance.

Of all the stages, in my opinion, the hardest to conquer are anger and depression. Let's face it, you have a lousy illness. You have every right to be angry and depressed. Your life is no longer what it once was and it is doubtful that it ever *will* be as it was.

Here's our suggestion to help you deal with these feelings: have yourself a private "pain and pity" party. Rail against your illness. Be VERY angry at it! Swear at it! Kick it and pummel it! DO IT! DO IT!

I SAID, *DO* IT! *NOW!*

(We'll wait.)

(hum-m-m-m-mmm-mmmm)

Okay. Are you done? Good. Now forget it. Get on with your life. Holding on to anger and depression will only serve to create an environment for pain and self-pity to flourish, which in turn will lead to more anger, deeper depression, and more pain. You don't need this.

Lose the anger. Lose the self-pity. Only then will you begin to be able to control your pain and start the healing process. During this process you will feel as if you are on an emotional roller coaster. You are angry because you aren't *you* anymore. You can't do everything you think needs to be done. You can't run the home, raise the children, hold down a full time job, and do volunteer work all at the same time. Why, sometimes you can't even walk and chew gum at the same time. You are angry, you're depressed, you're anxious — and — you're in pain.

HEATHER

Heather had everything a person could want — youth, intelligence, abundant energy, loving parents, a handsome young husband who adored her, and her whole life ahead of her. She held down two jobs and looked forward to entering college to earn a nursing degree.

In the performance of her job as a certified nursing assistant in home health care, Heather was treating a patient with an abscess that ruptured, spraying Heather with pus. Although Heather cleansed herself immediately, within two days of the incident she developed strep throat and scarlet fever. Although she was treated with antibiotics, Heather never really recovered. In retrospect, her doctors believe this incident eventually led to the diagnosis of CFS. It is still difficult for her to accept. "I'm too young to be this sick!" she would say.

Throughout the first meeting she spent with our support group, Heather cried. She didn't deserve this. She would say, "I'm too young to have this. I don't *want* to have it." She was full of anger, fear, and disbelief.

It was several months before Heather learned that you don't have to like a situation in order to accept it. The Thief is her enemy. She despises it, but now accepts it. Her life is not what she wants it to be, and probably never will be. Her illness has forced changes in her life and in the lives of her family. She understands that what she had planned for her life isn't likely to occur and realizes she must change her plans.

Heather's family wants to wrap her up in a cocoon and protect her. They must learn not to do too much for her and instead encourage her to do more for herself. Luckily, she discovered that she is stronger than either she or her family once thought. Her remissions are lasting longer and she is using the time to help others. She's taken on the leadership

of another support group and has accepted what life has in store for her.

Heather's story is a reminder to accept what is happening and focus on the things you *can* do, rather than what you can't. You can talk. To a friend, a pastor, a support group, a mental health professional, or your Aunt Mabel. No matter who you choose to vent to, you have made a *positive* decision.

If you decide to see a professional counselor, it's important to find one who believes in, and has had experience working with, fibromyalgia or chronic fatigue syndrome patients. You may ask how to determine whether or not a therapist has the experience you seek. It's simple — ask them. If a prospective therapist tells you s/he has lots of experience and can "cure" you, run away as fast as you can and stay as far away as possible. THERE IS NO CURE FOR CFS OR FIBROMYALGIA.

If you can't find a therapist who is experienced in treating fibromyalgia patients, try to find someone with an open mind who is willing to learn about your illness. Now, excluding your Aunt Mabel, what kind of a professional should you see?

You could see a psychiatrist, social worker, or a psychologist. Each has a different approach to your problem. Psychologists use many different forms of therapy to help their patients identify their problems and overcome them. Cognitive behavior therapy (CBT) is one therapy they may use. Psychologists are not medical doctors so they cannot prescribe medications.

A psychiatrist is a medical doctor specializing in mental health and can prescribe drugs. A psychiatrist encourages you to verbalize your problems so you can (hopefully) eventually figure out how to deal with and learn to solve them on your own. You may or may not need medications to reach your goals.

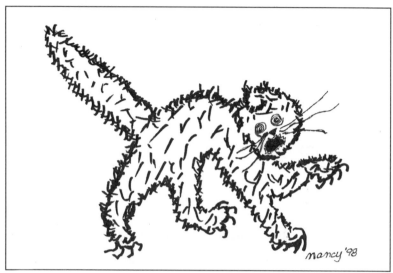

"Oh, S#&%!!!! HER PROZAC'S WORN OFF!"

Social workers are mainly problem solvers, adept at finding solutions. Social workers are more interested in what has happened and how to fix it than they are in *why* it happened. Their area of expertise is in bringing two or more parties together and resolving conflicts.

In a support group you will find a combination of all three of these professionals. Although they may not hold professional degrees, everyone in a support group *KNOWS, UNDERSTANDS,* and *BELIEVES* what you are experiencing. In a support group you are in the midst of experts, all with different personal experiences. They'll listen. They will allow you to vent (for a while), and then they will get down to the business of helping you. And you need not worry about confidentiality. In a support group, what is said in a room stays in that room.

You won't find all the answers you seek with any of these therapies overnight. It takes time. But you will find the help you need and deserve. So go ahead — give it a try. Let's talk.

17
SUPPORT GROUPS

No life is perfect. Learn to deal with what life hands
you and get on with the urgent business of living.
— *Nancy Fowler*

We cannot over-emphasize the importance of support groups. The first thing we tell people who ask for our help is "DON'T TRY IT ALONE!" You need help. Preferably from someone who has CFS/fibromyalgia.

If you are lucky, your health care team will know about a support group in your area. You can also try a Google search by typing in "fibromyalgia support groups" or "CFS support groups" and your home town into the Google search box. Check out the groups you find and see if they meet your needs — not every group will.

If you can't find a group, there is still something you can do — form your own group. One good place to start is to contact the National CFIDS Foundation for their booklet, "Support Group Guidelines: How to Organize a Self-Help Support Group for CFS/CFIDS/ME."

When you digest that information you can contact a local hospital or rheumatologist and talk to them about your desire to start a support group. Leave a flyer or business card with them. Ask them to post the information where others can see it and contact you. Ask local media (radio, local cable shows, and newspapers) to post free public service announcements. Don't be discouraged if the response is not as large as you want. It may take awhile to "get the word out" and it may be best to start out slow and get to feel comfortable in your new role. Contact local hospitals and/or libraries, lodges, etc. and ask if a place could be provided, at no cost, for your meetings to be held as a public service for the community. Choose a time that is convenient for you. You can't please everyone and since it is you who will be leading the group it is YOU who needs to be present.

As your group grows, you and your members can mold and form a format for what you want for your group. First of all, some semblance of order must be maintained. One or two must lead each meeting. Keep control and "lead" the conversation in the direction you desire. Allow people to "vent" if they need to, but then move on. Do not allow one person to monopolize the situation. Do not allow a "pity party" to form and take over. It doesn't help, people become discouraged and depressed, and no good is derived from it.

Having a co-leader helps reduce the stress because they undoubtedly have valid views and ideas to share and can take over the reins when "fibro-fog" and poor memory or recall strikes.

Speakers are always good to have, but limit their time. Don't allow them to take up the whole meeting. One of the biggest benefits of the group is the social time wit others who understand what is going on in each other's lives. We caution speakers that we will not allow them to sell or solicit at our meetings. That is our preference. You may feel differently.

We have found that you should not have speakers at every meeting. Sometimes it is more productive and helpful to have a "What's new with you? What do you do when…?" type of meeting.

Keep up on the latest research and stay informed. Don't be afraid to say, "I don't know — does anybody here know?" — or — "I'll try to find out and let you know at the next meeting."

We also keep an attendance sheet at each meeting and transfer each member to a master list which is kept by one or two (no more) of the leaders. This guarantees privacy to each member.

Over the years we have gathered a lot of information on our illness and hints on how to cope with it. We have put some of that information into a packet that we give, free of charge, to each new member.

When someone new comes to the meeting and asks if we can recommend someone for them to go to, for instance, a doctor, lawyer, psychologist, etc., we can help. We give out a form which we call a "Referral Rating Sheet" and ask every one to fill them out for every professional they have been to and ask them to give their honest opinion on them. (A sample of this form can be found in the Appendix, feel free to copy and use.) We INSIST that these forms remain unsigned as we feel anonymity is a MUST. We keep all these forms in one notebook and that notebook NEVER leaves the possession of ONE (and only one) of the leaders. We bring that book to each meeting so it may be examined then and there. We do not allow copies to be made of any of those completed forms.

Lastly, it may be best if you wait to start a support group until you are very comfortable and knowledgeable about your condition. When you decide to try being a support group leader, you MUST be ready physically and emotionally. You need to be comfortable and confident in your new role. Once you are ready the sky is the limit! You will be a blessing to those who come to you for help. It is also a good idea for you to contact other support group leaders to see how they operate. No matter how you choose to proceed, we only ask one thing of you — PLEASE do not give up! Support groups and people willing to be support group leaders are in short supply and are desperately needed. Don't give up for you are, and will be, providing a valuable service.

In conclusion, don't try to be the "know all — end all — lean on me at all times" kind of leader or I guarantee you will burn out. YOU need support, too! Seek it out if necessary. Accept it when it is offered. Don't forget the words in the song "We all need somebody to lean upon." Do not put unrealistic expectations on yourself...you are NOT God...you will not be perfect...you will not be successful 100% of the time, some people will be beyond your capabilities to help and you MUST accept that. And, remember this: You are human — you have your limits — you are sick too!

18
HUGS DON'T HAVE TO HURT

Do you not see that you and I are as the branches in one tree? With your rejoicing comes my laughter, with your sadness start my tears. Love, could life be otherwise?
— *Tzu Yeh*

The need for loving touches does not go away when you have The Thief. Everyone needs them. It does mean that the touches need to be more gentle.

Your sex life does not have to be a thing of the past. Intimacy is still possible and indeed desirable. But just as in other areas of your life, some planning and adjustments must often be made. For example, taking your pain medications so peak effectiveness will be reached at the time you plan to be making love. Get extra rest beforehand; take a warm, relaxing bubble bath. Plan for no interruptions — ship the kids off to grandma's; unplug the phone or turn off the ringer and let the answering machine take your calls. Hide the car. Put a sign in the window or on the door that says, "GO AWAY." (This *really* works, believe me!). Have plenty of lubrication ready, cuddle up together, and let nature take its course.

There's no need to anticipate the act of making love with fear and trepidation. Be gentle with each other. Experiment with different positions. Take your time. Let delicious anticipation mount and prolong the act. Learn or rediscover each other's erogenous zones. Touch and caress more. Be creative. Indulge in longer foreplay. Take it slow and easy.

Human beings are passionate, intelligent, and creative creatures. We are self-indulgent. We are aware that there are many ways to pleasure ourselves and each other. Go ahead and use your imagination! Remember that sexual desire is a normal emotion and it's just the two of you in that room. Having The Thief doesn't mean you have to miss out on the warm, loving, pleasant feeling of the "after-glow."

This is *not* meant to be a "how to" chapter, but more of a "let's try" chapter. It's a plea to you and your lover to not allow The Thief to rob you of the precious gift of physical love. The Thief has stolen too much already.

19
HUMOR

*You can always trust a person with chronic fatigue
syndrome or fibromyalgia to tell the truth. Even if she
remembered what was said, she probably won't
remember who said it or what it was about.*
— *Nancy Fowler*

Why include the subject of humor in a book about a serious, often debilitating, exasperating, and painful chronic illness? Because it is necessary to do so. My sense of humor has helped me cope with my illness, especially when fibro-fog strikes.

Why do you laugh? Because something tickles your funny bone, that's why.

How do you *feel* after a good laugh? You feel pretty good — at least much better than you did before. Laughter *is* beneficial, both psychologically and physiologically.

Laughter causes particular physiological changes to occur in your body. Your heart rate and respiration increases, which increases blood flow throughout your body, increasing oxygenation.

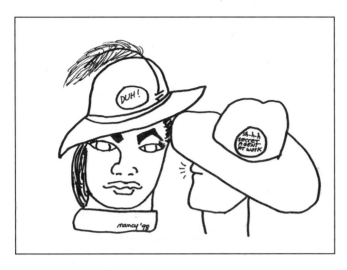

I do know *I* feel good after a good laugh. Often I feel my stress level decline and I can see a "problem" with new perspective. If I was in a bad mood before, I certainly can't go back to being in a bad mood again after a good laugh, no matter how much I might want to.

I recall a very stormy argument with my husband, about what I don't remember now, but during the silent treatment that followed, a rather humorous country song, "Wolf Creek Pass" came on the radio. As hard as we both tried, we couldn't hold it in, and the laughter came pouring out! The tense mood was broken and the path to reconciliation was started. So, laughter can definitely decrease stress and soothe emotions.

But how does laughter help you physically? I've learned at various medical conferences I've attended that laughter may help physically by elevating IgA levels which increases your immune response, lowering serum cortisol levels, increasing the number of killer T cells, and increasing tolerance to pain.

A very limited pilot study reported in *Mind/Body/Health Newsletter*, Volume 8, Number 2, 1999, found that people who have survived a heart attack and who laughed for at least 30 minutes daily required less medication, lowered their blood pressure, and were less likely to suffer a second heart attack. Although *not* a significant study in terms of size, the findings are tantalizing nonetheless.

Prestigious experts such as Dr. Donald Goldenberg, Dr. Anthony Komoroff, Dr. David Bell, and organizations such as the National CFIDS Foundation and the Massachusetts CFIDS Association firmly believe that "laughter is the best medicine," and I believe it, too. Maybe some serious, in-depth studies should be done.

As for me, I don't really care about the whys and wherefores; I just know that laughter makes me feel good. It helps me cope. It drives away depression. It makes me human. There is nothing I enjoy more than a good laugh — especially if it's on me.

Throughout this book you have encountered some examples of my own version of escapism. These cartoons are intended to make fun of our illness. Many of them are based upon actual events. The woman who forgot to remove her underwear before taking a shower — that really happened. And the husband who tells his wife that she wouldn't believe the headache he has — that happened. These are cartoons that people with The Thief in their life will understand and, hopefully, will bring at least a chuckle or two. And — this is completely unscientific — they will feel better and their pain will be decreased. For a while at least.

20
COPING STRATEGIES AND SURVIVAL TIPS

Never go to a doctor whose office plants have died.
— Unknown

It is our hope that this book will help you to cope effectively with The Thief and get on with your life. While there is no known cure, nor as yet any definitive treatment for The Thief, there are many changes you can incorporate into your lifestyle and mindset that will help you in the coping process. Here are some tips that have helped us. If you have any that have helped you but are not listed here, please let us know.

1. Accept the fact that you have an illness.
2. Learn all you can about your illness.
3. Work in partnership with your doctor(s).
4. Use common sense. If it hurts to do something, don't do it!
5. Reduce the stressors in your life.
6. Develop a positive attitude and refuse to be a victim.
7. Find a support group and become involved.

8. Become an advocate and educate others about your illness.

9. Don't assume all of your health problems are the result of CFS or fibromyalgia. Just because you have CFS or fibromyalgia doesn't mean you cannot have other, unrelated, sometimes serious illnesses.

10. Become organized. Be ready for those flares and when a flare does strike, don't fight it. Live by the old saying, "a place for everything and everything in its place." This is a defense mechanism, not the words of a neat freak. Being well organized lessens confusion when fibro-fog strikes and consumes less energy when cleaning up.

11. Recognize your limitations and don't apologize for them. Don't push yourself beyond your limitations.

12. Make life easier for yourself. Change your hairstyle if you find it difficult to maintain your current style. Dress comfortably and let fashion be damned! You have too much to contend with to be uncomfortable, too.

13. Discover and cultivate your sense of humor. Try to find the humor in any given situation. Learn to laugh at yourself.

14. Seek out and accept emotional and physical support when necessary.

15. If your home consists of two or more floors, save time and energy by placing a box on both the top and bottom stair. Whenever something needs to go up or down, place it in the box. The next person to go up or down can take the box with them.

16. Remember the Girl Scout motto and "Be Prepared." On your good days, when preparing a meal, make extra and freeze it for use on days when you are experiencing a flare.

17. Stock up on disposable plates, cups, and eating utensils to use when you are aren't feeling well.

18. Become a list maker. Keep a notebook handy to keep track of appointments, calls to make and what you want to say when you make the call, bills to pay, ideas you have, tasks you want to accomplish, etc. Don't laugh. This hint has saved me many times. (Don't forget the list when you go out!)

19. Don't apologize when you are unable to do something. You are the one who is ill and it's not your fault.

20. Unless the Board of Health has condemned your home, don't waste time or energy worrying about keeping it spotless. We have it on good authority that the Dust Police have officially disbanded and are no longer in existence. Besides, in a hundred years, who will know or care that your furniture was dusted and waxed and you were able to see your face in the woodwork? A clear, concise, descriptive warning about their fate should deter anyone from disturbing your dust. Spend your time in such quality pursuits as resting, reading, giggling with your child or grandchild, gossiping on the phone, etc.

21. Get a supply of large (10 x 13 inch) envelopes and label them with the names of friends and relatives. When you have something you want to give them or return to them, or an anecdote you want to relate — whatever — put it in the envelope. The next time you see that friend or family member you will have everything in readiness, and the words, "I know I have something for you but can't remember what," will not be uttered by you.

22. The hell with pride. Apply for and use a handicap-parking placard. And don't let anyone give you grief about using it.

23. Repeat after me, "It's okay to sit and rest awhile." Make it your mantra.

24. Develop a routine and try to stick to it.

25. Wear comfortable clothes and shoes. We joke that sweat suits are our "official fibro uniform" and I'm convinced that the person who invented permanent press should be awarded the Nobel Prize! Think of the enormous amounts of energy expended in keeping non-washable clothes clean. The cost, both physical and financial, to gather the clothes together, get to your car, drive to the cleaners, and then do it all over again when the clothes need to be picked up…WHEW! Tires me out just thinking about it!

26. Make sure you allow for plenty of extra time when you are going somewhere or planning a project, and when making appointments, don't make them for the first week of the month. Oftentimes you will find you have an appointment on the first day of the month only after you turn the page of the calendar.

27. It may sound silly, but have lots of night-lights going after dark. Having to get up many times at night, as we often do, it make sense to be able to see where we're going to avoid bumping our toes or tripping over something.

28. Keep a list of your medications and other important information near the phone. That's a given. But here is something that people rarely think to do — write down detailed instructions on how to get to your home and keep it with your medication list. If you need help from the police, fire department, or EMTs you are most likely going to be frightened and confused. If you do not

live in an area with Enhanced 911, your detailed instructions can be read to your rescuers so they can reach you faster.

29. Learn to establish priorities.

30. Repeat after me, "It's okay to sit and rest awhile."

31. Get some of those weekly pill containers with the days printed on the tops and pour your medications for a week or so at a time. You can also use them to keep your nighttime and your first-thing-in-the-morning medications beside your bed. Keep a pitcher of water and glass or a bottle of water nearby. This way, when you get ready to go to bed at night and realize you forgot to take your meds you won't have to go schlepping downstairs to take them. And, when you just can't drag yourself out of bed first thing in the morning, you will have your meds nearby so you don't have to be in a rush to get up.

32. Make your chores easier on yourself. I hate vacuuming! Hate it with a passion. But I'm also a person with dark rugs and light-colored, shedding dogs. Not a good combination, believe me. I got myself one of those lightweight carpet sweepers to use when my husband is not around to do the heavy vacuuming.

33. Do small jobs as they come up. Don't wait for things to pile up and become overwhelming.

34. Use voice mail or a telephone answering machine. Screen your calls and don't feel guilty about it.

35. Buy a wheeled utility cart so you can move things easily from room to room. Keep the cart stocked with frequently used housekeeping supplies such as furniture polish, cloths, etc. Keep a box on the cart for everything you pick up that isn't where it's

supposed to be such as toys on the floor or dishes in the bedroom.

36. If your house has multiple stories, keep duplicate cleaning supplies on each level.

37. Learn to meditate. Don't laugh, it works!

38. They had the right idea back when I was a kid; lots of stores had home delivery. Ask about home delivery where you shop. If it's available, take advantage of it when you just can't drag yourself out the door.

39. When running errands, help yourself and reduce stress by doing these things:

    a. Plan your route. WRITE IT DOWN.

    b. Make *detailed* lists. TAKE THE LIST WITH YOU.

    c. Take a day's supply of pills with you.

    d. Have a list of your medications with you at all times, along with your doctor's name and telephone number.

    e. Dress appropriately. If the weather is cold, *wear a hat* and gloves.

    f. Make sure someone knows where you are going and when you plan to be back.

40. Keep a notebook or battery-operated tape recorder in your car to make notes or dictate reminders to yourself. The tape recorder is especially handy when stopping and asking for directions. Just repeat the directions into the tape recorder as they are given to you. (This is very helpful when you are with someone who refuses to ask for directions himself!) There's another very handy use for it as well. I use my recorder to record some really snappy comebacks that I wish I had said but didn't!

41. As for personal hygiene, here are some suggestions:

    a. Shower or bath? They both have their advantages. A shower takes less energy but a nice, warm bath helps relax your tired, aching muscles.

    b. Sit while showering if possible.

    c. Sit on the toilet to dry off. This is especially handy if you are prone to dizziness. It also reduces muscle strain and helps you keep your balance.

    d. Dress and undress sitting down.

    e. Wash your hair in the shower instead of the sink. If you must wash your hair in the sink, provide support and stability by resting one leg on a stool to reduce pressure on your lower back.

    f. If it's time to shave, be sensible and use an electric razor — it's safer.

    g. If you just can't drag yourself to the shower and need to feel clean, try one of those commercial "wet wipes" or fill a spray bottle about ⅔ full of alcohol and ⅓ water along with about 2 tablespoons lemon juice. Spray on a cloth to wash up.

42. Buy a supply of folders or large envelopes and keep them together in one place. Use them to organize your mail: bills to be paid in one, correspondence in another, etc.

43. Pre-warm your bed at night by using an electric blanket or heating pad.

44. When you have to use a public restroom, be sure to use the handicapped toilet. These are raised higher than the others and take the strain off your legs.

45. Wear several layers of light clothing so you can remove and/or replace layers as temperature dictates.

46. Become a list maker. This is important. Don't rely on your memory.

47. Eat a healthy diet. Avoid caffeine, alcohol, and nicotine.

48. Practice stress reduction techniques.

49. Drink warm liquids and never use alcohol to "warm up."

50. Make time for yourself. SCHEDULE IT DAILY. Write it down! If it's not written down, you won't do it.

51. Take naps and rest whenever you feel the need.

52. Avoid any activity where you must keep your arms raised for any length of time, such as using a hair dryer.

53. Learn to say "NO!" when asked to do something that requires expending energy you need for yourself.

54. STOP BEFORE YOU DROP! I can't overemphasize this. Learn to listen to your body. Rest when you need to.

55. Have some soft, soothing music playing at low volume while you sit and relax.

56. Most important of all, have faith. Turn yourself over to a higher power. God will take care of you. He loves and understands you. Ask for a daily blessing that He will give you the strength to endure and accept that which you feel you cannot endure another day.

21
BEWARE OF FALSE PROPHETS

As if we were villains by necessity, fools by heavenly
compulsion.
— Shakespeare

It is said that a fool is born every minute and two to chase him. Sad, but true. Desperation plays a big part with our illness also. The more desperate you become for a cure or relief from your symptoms, the more willing you are to try anything and everything to secure relief, no matter how ridiculous, or even dangerous, it may be. It's a sad state of affairs when some people seek to take advantage of, and profit from, those who are most vulnerable. Our advice to you here is simple and direct — use your common sense.

IF IT SEEMS TOO GOOD TO BE TRUE, THEN IT IS.

How can you tell if something is too good to be true? How can you keep your hard-earned money in your pocket? How can you spot a lie? How can you tell if something will work? Just *when* will the alarm bells sound and whistles blow? All good questions.

As a rule, be suspicious of a remedy when:

- It promises a cure.

- It can only be purchased from one source and is promoted only by *paid* advertisement.
- It works for everything from curing headaches to growing green, green grass.
- The only proof of effectiveness is written testimonials from users.
- There is no list of ingredients or potential side effects, dangers, or drug interactions.
- You are told that this is the only thing you'll need, so you can throw away all the meds your doctor has prescribed and cancel the surgery that was recommended.
- It claims to work fast and keeps working permanently.
- It doesn't cost much.
- It makes claims of a "new and improved secret formula."

Trust that little voice whispering in your ear telling you to run away — fast! If it seems too good to be true, it usually is. However, if you do decide to try something "new and exciting and guaranteed to cure all your ills," please do these things *first*:

- Discuss it with your doctor and let him/her know you are going to try it.
- Continue with your established treatment regimen.

For safety reasons, make your family or a friend aware of the new treatment so they are able to observe your reactions and can check on you periodically.

When you're through trying this "modern miracle medicine" and are ready to admit you were taken, our government stands ready to help. To report your dissatisfaction, you can contact the Department of Health and Human Services, the U.S. Food and Drug Administration, the Federal

Trade Commission, and, for complaints about products that were promoted by mail, the United States Postal Service. You can find phone numbers online or in your telephone book under the heading United States Government.

But it's always best to use your common sense in the first place. Keep your money in your wallet and refuse to be taken in. We have given you the facts in this book. *THERE IS NO CURE (yet)!* And there is no such thing as a quick fix. If you are anxious to get rid of your hard-earned money, donate it a program that is researching your illness. The many people who donated to the research to discover the cause of CFS made a very wise investment that will benefit all of us.

22
SOCIETY AND THE THIEF

Beware of thy enemy once; of thy friends, a thousand times.
— Unknown

Because they hear the words, "You look so good!" or "You don't look sick!" and because they are told, "Your test results are all normal. I can't find anything wrong with you," the person with The Thief often experiences great frustration. Something *is* wrong! They feel rotten!

If they had some kind of visible physical impairment like a broken limb or arthritic deformity, the response of others would likely be quite different. People would most likely be sympathetic and helpful. The victim of The Thief, however, is often subjected to hostile stares, rude remarks, and interrogation by strangers, and sometimes friends and family members as well. This is especially evident when using a handicap parking placard or license plate to use a handicap parking spot.

Because of these attitudes, victims of The Thief become very sensitive to the spoken and unspoken criticisms of others. As a result, they feel unable to talk about their health concerns, fearing rejection and ridicule.

Interestingly, as victims of The Thief, we are often sought out and subjected to the endless recitations of the woes of others. We listen without complaining. Perhaps we have more empathy for the suffering of others. Regardless, the end result for us — STRESS — is something which we can ill-afford.

Our advice to victims of The Thief who have been belittled or criticized by supposed "friends" or family has always been this — spend as little time as possible with your detractors. When someone loves and cares for you, they believe in you and accept you as you are.

I realize it is not always easy advice to follow, but *you* come first now. You must learn to be selfish and consider *your* needs first. It's a matter of energy conservation, and you need to conserve what is left of yours.

NOW IN CASE YOU DIDN'T HEAR ME THE FIRST TIME OR NEGLECTED TO PAY ATTENTION, I'LL PUT IT SIMPLY — do *NOT* spend your valuable time with people who seem to do nothing but criticize you or who do not support you.

You've heard people say, "You make me sick!" Well, it's true; people *can* make you sick by causing you stress. Stay away from these people. Lay low for a while.

Sometimes you will find that family and friends don't seem to come around or call as much as they used to. That, too, is the fault of The Thief. You can't help it; your family and friends can't help it. You've made plans to go out, maybe to dinner and a movie. Then you have to back out, sometimes at the last minute, because you hurt too much or you're so exhausted you can't even think. The invitations dwindle and soon they stop entirely. No one wants to make plans, spend money, and then have you back out, or go along only to have to leave early. So they stop including you in their plans. This is understandable. It's sad, but understandable. You have The Thief to blame.

The up side of this (to us at least) is that we feel we've met some truly amazing people who have become our very good friends, all because of this damned illness. We cannot over-emphasize the importance of support groups and the strong, positive impact our support group has had in our lives.

There is a popular misconception regarding support groups of any kind. Many people feel that these groups serve no valid purpose and that the people who attend support meetings just sit around whining and crying and feeling sorry for themselves. Nothing could be further from the truth.

The primary reason for the existence of any support group is to provide help to the people who need it. That goal is accomplished by genuinely caring for and respecting all who seek the services of such a group. Often the people seeking out a support group view it as a last resort. These people are almost devoid of hope. Even though the pain they feel is real, they have begun to doubt themselves. This is probably the most vicious and dangerous aspect of The Thief — the self doubt.

Newcomers to a support group often feel that no one cares, no one believes them, and no one knows what they are experiencing. *THEY COULDN'T BE MORE WRONG!* Those in a support group do believe, care, understand, and know what the newcomer is going through, and because of this the support group can offer something truly precious — *hope.* Quite often after the first meeting, the newcomer will be in tears, realizing that *every* person in that meeting is going through the same thing and they truly do care and understand. They realize they are not alone and that they *can* and *will* survive this illness and its many challenges.

Many people with The Thief also turn to their spiritual beliefs for comfort. They discover or rediscover faith in a God who loves and cares for them and will help if He is asked. As with any wound, healing must start from within. You can't be healed on the outside if you are not whole and healed on the inside. Including God and prayer is a good way to start the healing process. God does not give us more than we can handle. You *can* and *will* learn to cope with your illness. You will survive it.

Helen's story shows how accepting her illness and taking responsibility for learning as much as possible about it turned into a mission to help others.

HELEN

Small, compact, full of energy. A spark plug. Helen was a dynamo. She was SUPERWOMAN! She was the original multi-tasker — an employer's delight! She could and would do the work of two or more people, and do it well.

She had always been like this. She had to be. It wasn't easy raising a large family, working outside the home, and keeping her house running, all to perfection. She even waited until she had some "free time" during a vacation to get the flu. That was ten years ago. She still has that "flu."

Helen spent years going from doctor to doctor, submitting to every test in the book. She spent thousands of dollars in the process. She needed answers, and she wouldn't stop until she got them.

Finally, after much research, she managed to put the pieces of the puzzle together and arrived at a diagnosis herself. The whole process had cost her dearly. Her health was in decline; her bank account dangerously low. It was hard to believe that she finally had an answer. Now she had to find a treatment. But first she had to have her diagnosis confirmed by her doctor.

Helen made an appointment with her rheumatologist and received the "official" CFS diagnosis — finally. But she got the feeling that she knew more about this illness than her doctor.

She hit the books again, researching at the library, on the Internet, and by telephone. She could not accept life as it was now. There had to be something to help her.

Helen was unhappy. She wanted things to be the way they were before. She liked to be able to plan something and know those plans would be followed through on. She liked things to be dependable, definite, and predictable and she knew CFS was unpredictable, limiting, uncontrollable, and unfixable. She was angry at The Thief for taking her life away. Her energy and drive were leaving her — her life would never be like it was before.

Despite her anger and without being consciously aware of it, Helen took her illness on. She fought it by not fighting it and not denying it.

She was born organized, so it seemed obvious to Helen that if she had this illness then others did too. She started a support group and discovered she was right about that. So many people answered her call she started another group. She left her "calling cards" (pamphlets, etc.) wherever she went. She made CFS her personal crusade.

When Helen wasn't researching on the internet, she was on the telephone calling anyone who could answer her questions. She learned many ways of coping with her illness and continues to live a fairly normal life. She does small jobs as they come up. She researches any new treatment she hears about and, if it sounds plausible, she'll try it. Many may think that's foolish, but she's driven to at least try.

Lately, she's been pushing herself too hard and has had to drastically curtail her activities. I can't say she's winning the battle against her illness, but she's not losing it either. She now spends many hours in bed, barely able to move. Barely able to express her anger and depression. We worry about her. We thank God for her.

23
SOCIAL SECURITY AND DISABILITY

Try first thyself, and after call in God, for the worker
God himself lends aid.
— Euripides

The United States of America is a wonderful place to live. A government *of* the people, *by* the people, and *for* the people, I firmly believe that our government *cares* for its people. And I believe her citizens truly care for each other.

Social Security is an example of this, and Medicare and Social Security Disability are only a part of this safety-net program for citizens suffering from disabling conditions.

I do *not* advocate that every person with The Thief quit working and apply for Social Security Disability (SSD). In fact, just the opposite is true. I *strongly* urge you to continue working for as long as you possibly can. It's good for you physically, psychologically, and financially.

Yeah, I know, there are some people who think that being able to stay home doing what they want with a monthly check coming in and

186

their health insurance paid for is the life they want to lead. And these people have learned how to manipulate the system and have learned how to lie very well. To those people I say, *SHAME ON YOU!*

Thankfully, more people work legitimately within the system than abuse it. People with The Thief are, as a general rule, want to work, have a good work ethic, and many exhibit Type-A personalities.

However, we must be realistic here. It is possible that there may come a time when you can no longer expect to continue working. For many of us that decision will come with great difficulty and will be put off for as long as possible. We make bargains with ourselves and with God. Eventually we must be truthful with ourselves and begin the process of applying for SSD. It is a gut-wrenching decision, and one that could lead to depression. We tell you this now so that you know what to expect and can prepare for it.

I have heard many people complain about our government and Social Security. I think in many cases it is just frustration and humiliation talking. I have found the Social Security Administration very helpful. I asked to be interviewed over the phone and they agreed. They helped me through every step of the process. Sure, I was turned down the first two times I applied, but I expected that. I was prepared. You can be too.

To begin the application process you have to make the call to Social Security at 1-800-772-1213. It's helpful to have all the information you need, but it is *not required* that you have it all to *start* the process. You will need your Social Security number and proof of age to start with. This is where the notebook with your medical history and information is essential. You need the names, addresses, and telephone numbers of every doctor you have seen, along with all the meds you take or have taken, all the treatments you have tried, and all the lab tests performed.

You also need to list *all* your symptoms and diagnoses, regardless of whether you consider them pertinent. List all of them.

Sit down and write a summary of where you worked and the type of work you did. *BE SPECIFIC.* Include everything you did *in descriptive detail* from the moment you set foot inside the workplace until the moment you left work. Write another summary of what you were able to do outside of the workplace. Again, be specific.

Next write another summary of what you are *now* able to do, again being specific. For example, what you are able to do now may look something like this: I wake up at 10:30 a.m. and lie in bed for twenty or so minutes, as I am unable to move without excruciating pain and fatigue. When I am able to get up, I go to the bathroom and brush my teeth. The effort wears me out so I go back to bed for a couple of hours until I feel I can once again force myself up to take a shower which once more leaves me exhausted. Etc., etc., etc. This may be a slightly

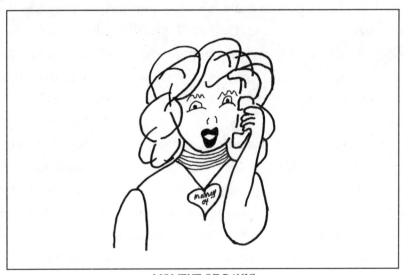

MOMENT OF PANIC
"Who am I calling? Why am I calling? AM I doing the calling or the answering??"

exaggerated description, but I think you get the idea.

There are many ways our government can help if you can no longer work, but what if you are still able to work with limitations? There are programs that can help you continue to work while disabled. There are programs to help with grocery bills or to learn a new skill. But you will never know what is available until you make that call.

Above all, be truthful. The person with The Thief should have no problem here, because in order to be a successful liar, you must to have a good memory, and the memory of a person with The Thief is not good at all. Why, sometimes we even have trouble remembering how to spell our own name!

24
"I'M F.I.N.E."

A strange and wonderful thing happens when you
believe in yourself, doubt is removed.
— Rodney Sherwood

How many times, when running into an old friend or acquaintance, have you been asked, "How are you?" It's a simple enough question. But, do they *really* want to know? Would their eyes glaze over or would they fall into a comatose state if you told them the truth? Would they even hear you if you launched into a litany of all your complaints?

Those of us who have The Thief know the answer: they *don't* really want to know. So in order to spare ourselves and others we've come up with an answer. We simply smile and say, "I'm F.I.N.E.!" Then our friend responds with a smile and says, "Great!" or something like that and goes on his/her way, oblivious to that fact that by F.I.N.E. we mean Frustrated, Irritated, Nauseated, and Exhausted!

By saying, "I'm F.I.N.E.!" we have given the answer they want to hear. They're satisfied, and the next time they see you they won't run in the opposite direction hoping that you didn't see them!

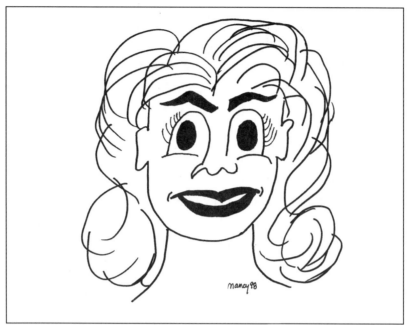

"Oh now, it can't be all that bad! After all, it's just Chronic Fatigue Syndrome. That means you're tired a lot, that's all. I mean...we all get tired."

How *well* I remember (before being diagnosed) running into an old friend that I hadn't seen for quite awhile. After the opening niceties, she innocently asked me how I was doing. Without thinking, I replied, "I've had a bad case of the flu for about six months now. I just can't shake it. If I have to think for a period of more than thirty seconds, I just *know* my head will explode. Some days it is all I can do to get out of bed and wash up. When I do, I have to go back to bed and rest for the remainder of the day because after I do that I am in so much pain and so worn out that I can't even remember my name. My doctors tell me there is nothing wrong with me. I've had every test in the book, and I think they made up a few just for me, and they all come back fine. I forget things. I think I have Alzheimer's. I never get out of the house; no one comes to visit or calls. I lost my job because I was always taking sick time and when I did work I had to leave early because I couldn't do my job. I am *seriously* thinking about suicide."

Did I get a positive, caring response from my friend (who now had that deer-in-the-headlights look)? Yeah, I did. She said, "Well, you look good! You don't look sick! See ya! Gotta go!"

I haven't seen or heard from her since. I wonder why.

Now that I have a diagnosis — a name for my miseries — everything is different. When someone asks me, "How are you?" my answer is, "I'm F.I.N.E., except for the fact that I have CFS (or fibromyalgia)."

The response I get now? "Oh. That's terrible! What a shame! My _____ (sister brother, aunt, friend, cousin) has that! It's just awful!"

Think I ought to try to contact my old friend? Nah! What was her name again?

EPILOGUE

Lisa and I wish to thank you very much for purchasing and reading our book. We hope that we have been of some help to you. This is a terrible illness we have. We urge you to learn as much as you can and to educate others about it. Most importantly, don't despair; believe in yourself, and never, *NEVER* ATTRIBUTE ALL OF YOUR HEALTH PROBLEMS TO THIS ILLNESS. Remember, just because you have chronic fatigue syndrome or fibromyalgia doesn't mean you can't get another illness. It's not fair, I know, but it's a fact.

Gentle hugz-z-z,

Nancy & Lisa

I REMEMBER YESTERDAY

STOP!...just stop…I can't take anymore.

I'm tired...so...tired, Just thinking's a chore

I want to find a corner to claim as my own

Tell the world to go away, and leave me alone.

Do this, do that…Come here, go there.

So many demands...Doesn't anyone care?

I can…no, I can't…If I could I would.

I have to…don't want to…Well, maybe I should.

Am I all right? Is it all in my head?

Is it normal to face each day full of dread?

Unsure, insecure…full of doubt…full of pain.

The hell with today, I want yesterday again.

Yesterday I *KNEW*…I was alive and secure.

Yesterday, I remember, I was confident, I was sure.

Dear God, if I'm good…I mean very, very good,

Will you answer my prayer? I know that you could.

Let me feel yesterday, let me feel whole.

Let me feel yesterday deep down in my soul.

I need your help to be me again.

I can't do it alone…Please…God…I'm in pain.

— *Nancy Fowler*

FURTHER INFORMATION

SUGGESTED READING

Fibromyalgia Explained, Pamphlet by Seacoast Chapter Support Group.

Fibromyalgia & Chronic Myofascial Pain Syndrome: Survival Manual, Devin Starlanyl.

Fibromyalgia Advocate, Devin J. Starlanyl.

From Fatigued to Fantastic, Jacob Teitelbaum.

Running on Empty, Katerina Berne.

When Muscle Pain Won't Go Away: Fibromyalgia, Gayle Backstrom and Dr. Bernard R. Rubin.

Chronic Fatigue Syndrome Cookbook, Mary Hale and Chris Miller.

Sick and Tired of Feeling Sick and Tired: Living with Invisible Chronic Illness, Paul J. Donoghue and Mary Elizabeth Siegel.

Fibromyalgia: A Comprehensive Approach, Miryam Ehrlich Williamson and David A. Nye.

Full Catastrophe Living: Using the Wisdom of your Body and Mind to Face Stress, Pain and Illness, Jon Kabat Zinn.

Osler's Web: Inside the Labyrinth of the Chronic Fatigue Syndrome Epidemic, Hillary Johnson.

Herbal Medicine, Dian Dincin Buchman.

Fibromyalgia and Chronic Myofascial Pain: A Survival Manual, Devin J. Starlanyl and Mary Ellen Copeland.

Relaxation and Stress Reduction Workbook, Martha Davis, Elizabeth Robbins Eshelman, Matthew McKay, and Patrick Fanning.

Freedom from Pain, Norman J. Marcus and Jean S. Arbeiter.

The Canary and Chronic Fatigue, by Majid Ali.

The Yeast Syndrome: How to Help Your Doctor Identify and Treat the Real Cause of Your Yeast Related Illness, John P. Trowbridge and Morton Walker.

Living with Chronic Illness, Cheri Register.

ONLINE INFORMATION

For those with Attention Deficit Disorder and FMS www.add-fibromyalgia.com

CENTERS FOR DISEASE CONTROL: for definitions, etc. www.cdc.gov

CFIDS site: publishes an online newsletter www.ourfm-CFIDSworld.org

CO-CURE: E-mails and articles (mostly from Britain): www.co-cure.org

FREE EMAIL ACCOUNT: www.myfibrosite.com

FIBRODOC.ORG: Information for your physician, massage therapist, or chiropractor, etc. www.fibrodoc.org

FIBROHUGS: Information and support: www.fibrohugs.com

FIBROMYALGIA NETWORK: Newsletter and website: www.fmnetnews.com

FIBROMYALGIA RESOURCE CENTER: Patient registry and doc find www.fmsresource.com

Massachusetts CFIDS/ME & FM Association: one of the oldest voluntary patient associations in the United States. www.masscfids.org/

MEDSCAPE: very credible web site for good medical information. They also publish an e-mail newsletter with current medical news www.medscape.com

MEN WITH FMS www.merlinean.com

MEN WITH FIBRO www.menwithfibro.com

MYALGIA.COM: herbal information www.myalgia.com

NATIONAL FIBRO AWARENESS CAMPAIGN: superb resource and publishers of the FMS magazine www.fmaware.org

NATIONAL FIBROMYALGIA PARTNERSHIP: publisher of quarterly *Fibromyalgia Frontiers* www.fmpartnership.org

PARTNERS AGAINST PAIN: free materials on pain, tips to control pain, links to pain support groups www.partnersagainstpain.com

PROHEALTH: Newsletter by e-mail, store, chat rooms, events, bulletin boards, discussion, clinical trials, great source of general information for fibromyalgia, CFS, and several other diseases. www.ProHealth.com

PUB MED: National Library of Medicine www.ncbi.nlm.nih.gov/PubMed/

REVOLUTION HEALTH: what works and what doesn't, rated by those who have tried them www.revolutionhealth/drugs-treatment

RX LIST: plain-English prescription information www.rxlist.com

SUICIDE/DEPRESSION: online therapy and mental health information www.metanoia.org/imhs

WEB MD: great source for general medical information www.webmd.com

OFFLINE INFORMATION

Fibromyalgia Aware Magazine: Call 714-921-0150 to subscribe, $35/year for print, $20/year on line.

Fibromyalgia Network Journal: national quarterly newsletter with information about coping, disability issues, insurance claims, treatment options, etc. $19/year. Contact by phone 800-853-2929, on the web www.fmnetnews.com or mail, PO Box 31750, Tucson, AZ 85751.

Fibromyalgia Frontiers: national newsletter with information on research, pain control, coping tips, medications, support groups, and upcoming seminars. Included with membership in the National Fibromyalgia Partnership. To join go to www.fmpartnership.org.

FMS Stretching Video: available from Fibromyalgia Information Foundation. www.myalgia.com.

The Forum: quarterly news magazine and excellent resource from the National CFIDS Foundation, 103 Aletha Road, Needham, MA 024920-3931. Comes with membership in the organization. www.ncf-net.org. 781-449-3535.

APPENDIX

DAILY DIARY

Today's Date: _____Day _____

Today I feel: Good____ Fair____ Poor_____

Today's Weather: Hot__ Warm__ Cool__ Cold__ Sunny__ Cloudy__

  Overcast__ Foggy__ Damp__ Rainy__ Snowy__ Windy__

A.M.: Weight_____ Temp _____BP_____ Sugar Level _____

P.M.: Weight_____ Temp _____BP_____ Sugar Level _____

Number of hours slept last night: ____ Sound? ____ Restless? ____

Naps taken today: How many? _____ Total hours _____

Regular medications taken today: (include vitamins, herbs, etc.)

Medication	Dose	Time	Results

Medications taken prn (as needed — e.g. aspirin for headache, etc.)

Medication	Dose	Reason	Time	Results

Physical Activity today: _____ Time spent on activity: _____

DIET:

Breakfast: _____ Lunch: _____

Supper: _____Snacks: _____

BODY MAP

Rate from 0 to 10 where 0 = no pain and 10 = the worst pain you can imagine. Mark the intensity at the location on the body map, e.g., 2 on the elbow.

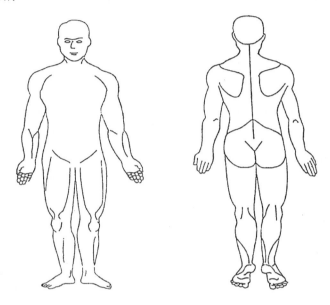

FEELINGS/SYMPTOMS TODAY:

FATIGUE	SUGAR CRAVINGS	BRITTLE NAILS
IRRITABILITY	SWEATING	ITCHING
NERVOUSNESS	HUNGER TREMORS	RASHES
DEPRESSION	PALPITATIONS	BLURRING VISION
INSOMNIA	PANIC ATTACKS	IRRITATED EYES
IMPAIRED MEMORY	FRONTAL HEADACHES	NASAL CONGESTION
POOR CONCENTRATION	OCCIPITAL HEADACHES	ABNORMAL TASTES
RESTLESS LEGS	GAS	RINGING EARS
LEG CRAMPS	BLOATING	NUMBNESS
DIZZINESS	CONSTIPATION	WEIGHT CHANGES
BLADDER INFECTIONS	DIARRHEA	DYSURIA
PUNGENT URINE		

ANESTHESIA PROTOCOL

"Recent research funded by the NCF that found ciguatera toxin being produced by a disease process in the body points to the danger of using any anesthesia that uses the sodium channel. Ciguatoxin affects the sodium channel function at the cellular level. Some anesthesiologists have had success blocking the sodium channel during anesthesia for ME/CFS patients.

"I would recommend that potentially hepatotoxic anesthetic gases *not* be used, including Halothane. Patients with Chronic Fatigue Syndrome are known to have reactivated herpes group viruses that can produce mild and usually subclinical hepatitis. Hepatotoxic anesthetic gases may then provoke fulminate hepatitis. Finally, patients with this syndrome are known to have intracellular magnesium and potassium depletion by electron beam x-ray spectroscopy techniques. For this reason I recommend the patient be given Micro-K using 10m Eq tablets, 1 tablet BID and magnesium sulfate 50% solution, 2 cc IM 24 hours prior to surgery. The intracellular magnesium and potassium depletion can result in untoward cardiac arrhythmias during anesthesia. For local anesthesia, I would recommend using Lidocaine sparingly and without epinephrine." — Paul R. Cheney, M.D., Ph.D., 1992

"Suggestions on anesthesia include using Diprivan as the induction agent along with nitrous oxide and isoflurane (Furane) as the maintenance agent. The ones to avoid are histamine releasers that include sodium pentothal as well as a broad group of muscle relaxants in the curare family, including Traceium and Mecacurium" — Patrick L. Class, M.D. 1996

Reprinted with permission of National CFIDS Foundation; Gail Kansky, President

RESOURCE, REFERRAL, AND RATING SHEET FOR PROFESSIONAL SERVICES

Please use this form for your *ANONYMOUS* appraisal of any professional you have had experience with (doctors, lawyers, physiatrists, therapists, etc.) This information will provide a valuable resource for support group members.

Name: ....

Profession: ....

Street address: ....

City: ....State: ......Zip: ....

Telephone: ....

Please use the space below to tell us something about your experience with this person (Was s/he: Supportive? Caring? Knowledgeable about your problem? Rude? Opinionated? Pleasant? Diagnosis only? Second opinion only? Willing to work with you? Helpful or not?

SPECIAL NOTES: ....

....

....

REGARDING THIS INDIVIDUAL, I WOULD

☐ Recommend this person

☐ NOT recommend this person

☐ Definitely AVOID this person

ADDITIONAL COMMENTS: ………………………...………………….

………………………………………………………………………….

………………………………………………………………………….

………………………………………………………………………….

Feel free to copy this form for your support group if you wish. The person filling it out MUST NOT sign it. ANONYMITY IS A MUST.

GLOSSARY OF TERMS

allergist — a medical professional specializing in allergies and allergic reactions

anorexia — the inability or unwillingness to eat

burnout — to become physically and emotionally unable to continue to function at a given task

CFIDS — chronic fatigue and immune dysfunction syndrome

CFS — chronic fatigue syndrome

cognitive — relating to or involving thinking, perception, reasoning, remembering, and processing information

constricted — to become narrow or smaller

contagious — "catchy"; spreading (such as illness) from one person to another

dilated — to become enlarged or bigger

electrolytes — chemical substances in the body that are responsible for the optimal functioning of all cells and for the transmission of nerve impulses

endometriosis — abnormal growth of uterine tissue causing increased menstrual bleeding, often with pelvic pain and discomfort

erogenous — erotic or sexual feelings or sensations

exacerbation — to become worse or more severe; a flare

familial — tending to occur more frequently in families; genetic predisposition

fibro-fog — also known as "brain fog"; difficulty remembering and assimilating information

fibromyalgia — a disease characterized by pain in the muscles and tissues that surround them

F.I.N.E. — Frustrated, Irritated, Nauseated, Exhausted or Frustrated, Irritated, Nothing works, Everything stinks

flare — a recurrence or worsening of symptoms

FM or FMS — fibromyalgia; fibromyalgia syndrome

foreplay — sexual stimulation engaged in before intercourse

GWS — Gulf War Syndrome

homeostasis — the ability of the body to maintain normal functioning while changes are occurring within the body

hyper — increased or more

hypersomnia — excessive sleep

hypertonicity — a state of excessive muscle tone or tension

hypo — decreased or less

hypochondria — excessive concern about one's health; imagining symptoms that aren't there or blowing symptoms out of proportion, convincing oneself that symptoms are serious and life threatening

hypoxia — when the body starves for oxygen; caused by conditions such as dehydration, heart and lung diseases, and living at a high altitude

IBS — irritable bowel syndrome; bouts of diarrhea and or constipation

immunologist — a medical doctor specializing in immune disorders and immune responses, especially allergies and hypersensitivities

infectious disease specialist — medical professional who specializes in treating communicable diseases insomnia — the inability to get to sleep, remain asleep, or attain restorative sleep

KISS — an acronym for Keep It Simple, Stupid and this author's philosophy; meaning get back to the basics

libido — sexual desire

MVP — mitral valve prolapse; a disorder of the heart that may cause a murmur

MCS (multiple chemical sensitivities) — having reactions to many different chemicals/drugs that may not have caused problems in the past

NCP or nursing care plan — a plan of action or treatment that nurses use when organizing the care of a patient

panic or anxiety attack — sudden onset of extreme and unreasonable fear or anxiety

PMS (pre-menstrual syndrome) — a variety of unpleasant symptoms (headache, bloating, irritability, etc.) that can occur one to two weeks before onset of menses

polycythemia — when the body makes more cells to answer the need for more oxygen due to a condition called hypoxia

PWF/C/ME/TT — **P**erson **W**ith: **F**ibromyalgia/**CFS**/**M**yalgic **E**ncephalomyelitis/**T**he **T**hief

REM (rapid eye movement) — a stage of sleep when the brain is quite active, during which there is rapid movement of the eyes, usually associated with a vivid dream state

remission — a period of time when symptoms disappear and you feel normal

restless legs syndrome (RLS) — a creepy, crawly sensation in the legs; usually not painful but extremely uncomfortable; relieved by walking or moving the legs

rheumatologist — a medical doctor specializing in conditions of the
joints and connective tissues such as found in arthritis, fibromyalgia,
etc.

support group — a group of people who meet to discuss a particular
condition or problem they have in common; the purpose of which is
to offer each other emotional support, define and solve problems,
and offer solutions and/or answers to problems encountered

syndrome — a collection of symptoms or features which occur together
and characterize a specific illness or abnormality

wax and wane — to increase and then decrease in intensity, comes and
goes, as in the phases of the moon

WNL — within normal limits; especially when referring to normal lab
test results

BIBLIOGRAPHY

Much of the information put forth in this book was gathered during the course of our professional work and training and the experience of living with the disease for many years. However, due to this illness, there were times when we did not trust our memories and felt it prudent to re-check or find additional information from the sources listed here:

Brooks, Barbara, Nancy Smith, Andrew Guthrie, Robert Hallowitz. *CFIDS — An Owner's Manual*, Silver Springs, MD: BBNS Publishing, 1990.

Buchfuhrer, Mark J., Wayne Hening, Clete Kushida. *Restless legs syndrome: Coping with sleepless nights,* St. Paul, MN: AAN Enterprises, 2007

Hebert, Raymond G. *Florence Nightingale: Saint, reformer or rebel?* Malabar, FL: Robert Kreiger Publishing, 1981. A collection of essays:

"Heroine of Modern Progress," Elmer C. Adams and Warren Dunham Foster (p.107);

"Florence Nightingale: Rebel with a Cause," by Charlotte Isler (p.181)

Lewis, Shawn M. and John Cox Collier. *Medical-surgical nursing: Assessment and management of clinical problems.* New York: Mosby, 1983.

Miller, Benjamin F. and Claire Brackman Keane. *Encyclopedia and dictionary of medicine, nursing, and allied health*, 7th Ed. New York: WB Saunders, 2007.

Mindell, Earl. *Earl Mindell's New Herb Bible.* Simon & Schuster/Fireside; 1992.

The Forum, Needham, MA: National CFIDS Foundation.

Chronic fatigue syndrome: A primer for physicians and allied health professionals, Quincy, MA: Mass CFIDS Association.

Health Watch Magazine, Santa Barbara, CA: ProHealth, Inc.

Rahe, Richard. *Life changes scaling for the 1990s,* Reno, NV.

Sleep walkers, Rochester, MN: Restless Legs Syndrome Foundation.

Woodham-Smith, Cecil. *Florence Nightingale, 1820 – 1910.* New York, NY: McGraw-Hill, 1951.

Diagnostics — patient preparation; interpretation; sources of error; post-test care, Nurses Reference Library — Nursing 82 Books. Springhouse, PA: Intermed Communications, Inc.

American Metabolic Laboratories, 1818 Sheridan St., Suite 102, Hollywood, FL 33020.

Healthwise, PO Box 1989, Boise, ID 83701

Web sources: www.webmd.com, www.howstuffworks.com, and www.rlshelp.org.

INDEX